T0325508

Focal Therapy in Prostate Cancer

Focal Therapy in Prostate Cancer

EDITED BY

Hashim U Ahmed MRCS, BM, BCh, BA(Hons)

Division of Surgery and Interventional Science
University College London
London, UK

Manit Arya FRCS, FRCS(Urol)

Department of Urology
University College London
London, UK

Peter Carroll

Department of Urology
University of California
San Francisco, CA, USA

Mark Emberton

Division of Surgery and Interventional Science
University College London
London, UK

⊛WILEY-BLACKWELL

A John Wiley & Sons, Ltd., Publication

Registered office: John Wiley & Sons, Ltd, The Atrium, Southern Gate, Chichester, West Sussex, PO19 8SQ, UK

Editorial offices: 9600 Garsington Road, Oxford, OX4 2DQ, UK
The Atrium, Southern Gate, Chichester, West Sussex, PO19 8SQ, UK
111 River Street, Hoboken, NJ 07030-5774, USA

For details of our global editorial offices, for customer services and for information about how to apply for permission to reuse the copyright material in this book please see our website at www.wiley.com/wiley-blackwell

Library of Congress Cataloging-in-Publication Data
Focal therapy in prostate cancer / edited by Hashim U. Ahmed ... [et al.].
     p. ; cm.
  Includes bibliographical references and index.
  ISBN-13: 978-1-4051-9649-9 (hardcover : alk. paper)
  ISBN-10: 1-4051-9649-1 (hardcover : alk. paper)
  1. Prostate–Cancer–Surgery. 2. Cancer–Diagnosis. I. Ahmed, Hashim Uddin.
  [DNLM: 1. Prostatic Neoplasms–surgery. 2. Ablation Techniques. 3. Neoplasm Staging. WJ 762]
  RC280.P7F63 2012
  616.99′463–dc23   2011015318

A catalogue record for this book is available from the British Library.

This book is published in the following electronic formats: ePDF 9781444346862; Wiley Online Library 9781444346893; ePub 9781444346879; Mobi 9781444346886

Set in 10/13 pt Meridien by Aptara® Inc., New Delhi, India
Printed in Singapore by Ho Printing Singapore Pte Ltd
1   2012

Contents

Contributor List

Hashim U. Ahmed MRCS, BM, BCh, BA (Hons)
MRC Clinician Scientist in Uro-Oncology
Clinical Lecturer in Urology
Division of Surgery and Interventional Sciences
University College London
London, UK

Clare Allen MD, FRCR, BM, BCh
Consultant Radiologist
Department of Radiology
University College London Hospitals NHS
Foundation Trust
London, UK

Nimalan Arumainayagam MD
Specialist Registrar in Urology
Division of Surgery and Interventional Sciences
University College London
London, UK

Dean C. Barratt PhD
Senior Lecturer in Medical Image Computing
UCL Centre for Medical Image Computing
University College London
London, UK

Al B. Barqawi MD, FRCS
Associate Professor of Surgery/Urology
Director of Prostate Cancer Fellowship Program
Division of Urology
University of Colorado Denver School of
Medicine
Aurora, CO, USA

Winston E. Barzell MD, FRCS, FACS
Clinical Assistant Professor
FSU College of Medicine
Urology Treatment Center
Sarasota, FL, USA

Nacim Betrouni PhD
INSERM
University of Lille Nord de France
Lille, France

Michael D. Brundage MSc, FRCPC, MD
Professor
Department of Oncology and Department of
Community Health and Epidemiology
Queen's University; and
Radiation Oncologist
Cancer Centre of Southeastern Ontario
Kingston, ON, Canada

Director
Division of Cancer Care and Epidemiology
Cancer Research Institute
Queen's University
Kingston, ON, Canada

Peter R. Carroll MD, MPH
Professor and Chair
Department of Urology
UCSF Helen Diller Family Comprehensive
Cancer Center
University of California, San Francisco
San Francisco, CA, USA

Pierre Colin MD
Chef de clinique Assistant
Department of Urology
CHRU Lille, University of Lille Nord de France
Lille, France

Matthew Cooperberg MD, MPH
Assistant Professor
Department of Urology
UCSF Helen Diller Family Comprehensive
Cancer Center
University of California, San Francisco
San Francisco, CA, USA

E. David Crawford MD
Professor of Surgery/Urology/Radiation
Oncology
Head Urologic Oncology
E. David Crawford Endowed Chair in Urologic
Oncology
University of Colorado, Denver
Aurora, CO, USA

Cole Davis MD
Clinical Oncology Fellow
Department of Urology
UCSF Helen Diller Family Comprehensive
Cancer Center
University of California, San Francisco
San Francisco, CA, USA

**Nandita M. deSouza BSc, MBBS, MD,
FRCP, FRCR**
Professor of Translational Imaging
Institute of Cancer Research and Royal Marsden
Hospital
London, UK

**Mark Emberton FRCS (Urol), FRCS,
MD, MBBS, BSc**
Professor of Interventional Oncology and
Honorary Consultant Urological Surgeon
Division of Surgery and Interventional Science
University College London
London, UK

NIHR UCL/UCH Comprehensive Biomedical
Research Centre
London, UK

Deb Feldman-Stewart PhD
Cognitive Psychologist
Division of Cancer Care and Epidemiology
Cancer Research Institute
Queen's University
Kingston, ON, Canada

Professor
Department of Oncology
Queen's University
Kingston, ON, Canada

Elizabeth M. Genega MD
Staff pathologist
Beth Israel Deaconess Medical Center
Boston, MA, USA

Assistant Professor
Harvard Medical School
Boston, MA, USA

Michael S. Gee MD, PhD
Assistant Radiologist
Abdominal Imaging and Interventional
Radiology
Massachusetts General Hospital
Harvard Medical School
Boston, MA, USA

Assistant Professor
The University of Texas
MD Anderson Cancer Center
Houston, TX, USA

**David J. Hawkes PhD, CPhys,
FMedSci, FREng, FInstP, FIPEM**
Director of the UCL Centre for Medical Image
Computing
University College London
London, UK

Mukesh G. Harisinghani MD
Director of Abdominal MRI
Associate Professor of Radiology
Department of Radiology
Harvard University
Boston, MA, USA

Timothy K. Ito
Resident in Urology
Division of Urologic Oncology
Department of Urology
New York University Langone Medical Center
New York, NY, USA

Rajat K. Jain
Resident in Urology
New York University Langone Medical Center
School of Medicine
New York, NY, USA

Irving Kaplan MD
Assistant Professor Radiation Oncology
Harvard Medical School
Boston, MA, USA

Beth Israel Deaconess Medical Center
Boston, MA, USA

**Alex Kirkham BM, BCh, FRCS,
FRCR, MD**
Consultant Radiologist
Department of Radiology
University College London Hospitals NHS
Foundation Trust
London, UK

Laurent Lemaitre MD, PhD
Professor
Department of Radiology
University of Lille Nord de France
Lille, France

Paul D. Maroni MD
Assistant Professor
Division of Urology
Department of Surgery
University of Colorado School of Medicine
Aurora, CO, USA

Caroline M. Moore MD, MRCS (Ed)
Clinical Lecturer in Urology
University College London and University
College London Hopsitals NHS Trust
London, UK

Vladimir Mouraviev MD
Clinical Fellow Instructor
Urology Division
Department of Surgery
University of Cincinnati
College of Medicine
Cincinnati, OH

Anwar Padhani MBBS
Consultant in Radiology
Paul Strickland Imaging Centre
Mount Vernon Cancer Centre
Northwood, Middlesex, UK

Rodrigo Pinochet MD
Urologic Oncology Fellow
Memorial Sloan-Kettering Cancer Center
New York, NY, USA

Associate Instructor
Department of Urology
Pontificia Universidad Catolica de Chile
Santiago, Chile

Louis L. Pisters MD
Professor of Urology
The University of Texas MD Anderson Cancer
Center
Houston, TX, USA

Thomas J. Polascik MD, FACS
Director of Urologic Oncology
Duke Cancer Institute
Duke University Medical Center
Durham, NC, USA

Philippe Puech MD, PhD
Associate professor of Radiology
CHRU Lille
University of Lille Nord de France
Lille, France

INSERM
University of Lille Nord de France
Lille, France

Neil Rofsky MD
Professor of Radiology
Department of Radiology
Beth Israel Deaconess Medical Center
Boston, MA, USA

Sophie F. Riches MPhys Msc
Clinical Physicist
Institute of Cancer Research and Royal Marsden
Hospital
London, UK

Ulrich Scheipers PhD
TomTec Imaging Systems GmbH
Unterschleissheim, Germany
Ruhr-University Bochum, Bochum, Germany

Katsuto Shinohara MD
Helen Diller Family Chair in Clinical Urology
Professor, Department of Urology and Radiation
Oncology
University of California, San Francisco
San Francisco, CA, USA

Samir S. Taneja MD
James M. Neissa and Janet Riha Neissa
Associate Professor of Urologic Oncology
Director, Division of Urologic Oncology
Department of Urology
GU Program Leader, New York University
Cancer Institute
New York University Langone Medical Center
New York, NY, USA

Chief
Urology Section
Veterans Administration
New York Harbor Healthcare System
(Manhattan campus)
New York, NY USA

Nina Tunariu MD
Specialist Registrar in Radiology
Institute of Cancer Research and Royal Marsden
Hospital
London, UK

Arnauld Villers MD, PhD
Professor in Urology
Department of Urology
CHRU Lille, University of Lille Nord de France
Lille, France

John F. Ward MD, FACS
Assistant Professor
Department of Urology

The University of Texas
MD Anderson Cancer Center
Houston, TX, USA

Thomas M. Wheeler MD
Harlan J. Spjut Professor and Chair
Department of Pathology and Immunology
Baylor College of Medicine
Houston, TX, USA

Preface to the first edition

The diagnostic and therapeutic landscape of prostate cancer is one of the most exciting areas of medical research in our modern age. Very few conditions or diseases have caused as much controversy and debate in the medical and popular literature. The manner in which we currently diagnose and treat prostate cancer seems to lead to ever increasing cost to the individual patient, to his family, and to healthcare systems in general, but with great uncertainty over the benefits. The entire pathway has come into question, based as it is on inherent inaccuracy and lack of precision in locating, targeting, and treating the malignant tumor. Almost all other solid organ cancers rely on visualizing the cancer, sampling it accurately, and delivering therapy only to that area which requires it.

Focal therapy in prostate cancer supports a similar, albeit belated, paradigm shift. Such a change relies on accurate imaging, accurate biopsy, and accurate destruction of the cancer while minimizing collateral damage and preserving as much normal tissue as possible. What are the benefits? We may have an isoeffective treatment that carries less harm to the individual man in a more cost-effective way that benefits society. The challenges are tremendous—locating cancers in a walnut-sized organ is not easy—ablating areas to millimeter accuracy and ensuring the remainder of the tissue does not develop new cancers which progress into life-threatening disease. This book is written by international experts at the forefront of imaging and focal therapy of prostate cancer and will provide the reader with a comprehensive scientific approach to the aspirations and challenges of focal therapy.

Hashim U. Ahmed
Manit Arya
Peter Carroll
Mark Emberton
November 2011

Is there a role for Focal Therapy in Localised Prostate Cancer?

CHAPTER 1

The Rationale for Focal Therapy of Prostate Cancer

Cole Davis MD, Matthew Cooperberg MD MPH, and Peter R. Carroll MD MPH

Department of Urology, UCSF Helen Diller Family Comprehensive Cancer Center, University of California, San Francisco, San Francisco, CA, USA

Introduction

The goals of cancer therapy are either to prevent, cure, or control disease while minimizing the side effects of treatment. One must balance the number of life years gained (quantity) with the morbidity of a given treatment technique (quality). The ultimate goal is to match treatment type with the biological aggressiveness of the disease in an individual patient. A difficult initial hurdle is predicting disease aggressiveness. Nomograms and other risk-prediction instruments incorporating multiple pathologic, laboratory, and clinical measures have become the cornerstone in prostate cancer risk assessment. Accurate risk assessment guides treatment. In contemporary practice there is a continuing movement toward maximizing survival while minimizing morbidity.

This movement is seen clearly when examining the increasing use of laparoscopic and, more recently, robot-assisted laparoscopic techniques in the treatment of prostate and renal cancers as well as conformal and intensity-modulated radiation therapy (IMRT), cryotherapy, brachytherapy, and experimental modalities such as high-intensity focused ultrasound (HIFU) and photodynamic therapy in the treatment of prostate cancer. Minimally invasive techniques that deliver therapy to the cancer alone, with a margin of normal tissue, are attractive since the risks of local progression and thus metastasis are, at least in theory, decreased compared to surveillance, while the morbidity associated with radical resection or whole-organ ablation decreased.

Focal Therapy in Prostate Cancer, First Edition. Edited by Hashim U Ahmed, Manit Arya, Peter Carroll and Mark Emberton.
© 2012 Blackwell Publishing Ltd. Published 2012 by Blackwell Publishing Ltd.

The therapeutic dilemma

The morbidity associated with radical prostatectomy and radiotherapy is well described and is primarily a result of treatment effects on adjacent structures [1]. Overall, each of the whole-gland radical treatments can be associated with significant morbidity. Radiotherapy causes short-term moderate bowel and urinary toxicity in almost 50% with most having limited toxicity. However, 5–20% with bowel toxicity have long-term persistence. Select surgical series report as high as 27% risk of chronic urinary symptoms. Both radiotherapy and surgery have a near 50% reduction in sexual function, though the reports are widely variable. Additionally, newer techniques and increasing refinement in technology have shown very little change in the toxicity profiles [2].

Therefore, minimally invasive techniques applied to discreet tumor areas, rather than the whole gland, stand to modify treatment impact the most with regard to urethral, rectal, and cavernosal nerve injury. Additional advantages could include reduced hospital stay and earlier return to work. Prostate cancer is biologically unique given the indolent nature and protracted natural history of many lesions. This demands individualized treatment decisions that include active surveillance or active treatment currently in the form of whole-gland therapy. Although the trend is changing in recent years as more compelling data becomes available, few patients elect to defer initial treatment. Between 1989 and 2008, 11,892 men with localized prostate cancer were registered in the CaPSURE multi-institutional database, and of those, only 810 (6.8%) elected to defer treatment and be managed with watchful waiting or active surveillance [3]. The rationale for use of minimally invasive therapies must be based on the following principles:

1 The technique offers similar disease control compared to the current options.
2 It is less morbid.
3 It offers improved outcomes compared to patients managed conservatively.
4 The technique is cost effective.

Prostate cancer has significant mortality worldwide, yet has an incidence-to-mortality ratio of 8.6 in the United States, 3.0 in the United Kingdom, and 1.2 in Africa [4]. Such differences may reflect many factors, one of which is screening rates. This is supported by multiple autopsy series showing that 30–40% of men suffering nonprostate cancer related deaths harbor prostate cancer [5]. Additionally, incidental prostate cancer is found in 23–45% of men undergoing cystoprostatectomy for the management of bladder cancer.

The difficult choices faced by men who have localized prostate cancer are further confounded by the findings from the recent publication of the third interim analysis from the European Randomized Study of Screening for Prostate Cancer (ERSPC). This demonstrated a reduction in prostate cancer specific mortality from PSA screening and treatment [6]. However, the healthcare policy implications of screening need to be tempered. First, a randomized controlled study in the United States has shown no difference between PSA screening and control [7], although the control arm had a high degree of contamination since many men had already undergone a PSA test prior to enrolment. Second, there are considerable harms associated with a screening strategy. These include overtreatment and treatment-related harms. The ERSPC showed that 1410 men need to be screened and 48 diagnosed and treated in order that one prostate cancer related death is avoided over a 9-year interval. Overtreatment becomes less of a problem if the treatment is cost effective and associated with very low rates of harm, while eliminating potentially high-risk disease.

Cost

The cancer-attributable costs associated with the first 6 months of treatment in 1999 demonstrated that radical prostatectomy cost $8113, external beam radiotherapy cost $6116, and brachytherapy cost $7596 [8]. Another study from the same time period found mean hospital charges of $5660 for radical prostatectomy compared to $4150 for cryotherapy. Most of the cost savings for cryotherapy arise from hospitalization costs of $2348 for radical prostatectomy and $682 for cryotherapy [9]. Most cost analyses do not take into account lost productivity from multiple treatment visits required for radiation therapy or postoperative visits and urethral catheter time associated with surgery. Costs for newer forms of radiation such as IMRT and proton therapy are higher. Insurers and public interest groups are paying more attention to the costs of care in conjunction with their utility and wide variation in application [10,11]. Minimally invasive interventional techniques delivering focal therapy may have the advantage of being performed in a single, outpatient setting with fewer downstream costs of dealing with side effects, but this may need to be balanced with the rate of salvage therapies in the event of failure.

Conservative management

Active surveillance with the potential for delayed therapy must incorporate several elements:
1 Markers for disease progression are reliable.
2 Patients are compliant.

3 The cancer will not progress at a speed exceeding follow-up windows.

4 Treatment at the time of progression is effective.

5 Patients accept the potential anxiety associated with untreated cancer.

A meta-analysis including 828 patients on surveillance protocols found the risk of metastasis at 10 years after diagnosis in those with well-differentiated tumors to be 19% and cancer-specific mortality 13% [12]. Albertsen and colleagues have shown that many men with prostate cancer die of other diseases. Further, those with low-risk disease (well-differentiated tumors) managed conservatively can expect 10-year prostate cancer specific mortality of 8.3% [13]. Other studies suggest that men with prostate cancer may be at higher risk. Johansson et al. showed that cancer-specific survival dropped from 79% to 54%, as patients managed conservatively were followed past 15 years [14]. In addition, the Scandinavian prostate cancer group randomized trial of patients with localized prostate cancer in the pre-PSA era treated by radical prostatectomy or watchful waiting, revealed significant relative risk reductions in overall mortality, prostate cancer specific mortality, metastasis, and local progression in the former group. However, the benefit to treatment was seen in those less than 65 years of age. In addition, the patients in this trial were notably different than those currently detected with aggressive screening in the United States. For instance, only 12% had T1c disease and 20% had an initial PSA ≥ 20 ng/mL [15].

In the Toronto active surveillance cohort of 450 men overall survival was 78.6%. The 10-year prostate cancer actuarial survival was 97.2%. Overall, 30% had been reclassified as higher risk and offered definitive therapy [16]. The UCSF active surveillance series used stricter criteria and reflected a secondary treatment rate of 24% at 3-year median follow-up, although 37% met criteria for progression and 12% elected treatment without evidence of disease progression [17]. None have died in the UCSF series at a median follow-up of 3.6 years.

Minimally invasive therapies

Minimally invasive interventional techniques have been applied to whole-gland therapy for many years in order to find a middle ground between active surveillance and radical surgery or radiotherapy. The earliest such technique introduced for prostate cancer was radium brachytherapy in 1915. Another percutaneous technique is whole-gland cryotherapy. It shares many similar advantages with brachytherapy. Early outcomes using cryotherapy were worrisome with major complications reported such as urethrocutaneous and rectourethral fistula. Refinements in monitoring, urethral warming, and probe technology have brought about resurgence in interest in cryotherapy. A prospective randomized trial comparing cryoablation to external beam radiotherapy found near equivalent disease-free survival at 8 years and a significantly higher negative biopsy rate in those managed with cryoablation [18]. Katz et al. reviewed 5-year biochemical-free survival among patients treated with brachytherapy, conformal radiotherapy, radical prostatectomy, and whole-gland cryoablation in different series. When stratified according to low-, medium-, and high-risk disease, cryotherapy was equivalent to other modalities for low- and medium-risk patients and superior for high-risk patients [19]. The major disadvantage to whole-gland cryotherapy is the morbidity profile, most notably with regard to erectile dysfunction (approaching 100% in the whole-gland setting). Third generation, prostate cryoablation techniques have been in use since 2000 and have shown lower complication rates compared to previous techniques except for impotence. Reported complications include bladder outlet obstruction 3–21%, tissue sloughing 4–15%, and impotence 40–100% [20].

Other whole-gland techniques include HIFU and vascular-targeted photodynamic therapy (VTP). Early studies have yielded mixed results regarding efficacy and morbidity for these modalities [21]. For instance, HIFU whole-gland therapy seems to have incontinence rates (requiring pad usage) of less than 1%, impotence rates are still 20–50% [22]. However, application in a focal setting for well-selected patients may prove highly beneficial.

Focal therapy—the middle way?

Currently, minimally invasive modalities are receiving considerable interest applied as focal, rather than whole-gland, therapy [23,24]. Focal therapy involves the local application of therapy to a specific focus with a margin of normal tissue. Therapy can be applied ranging from a small focus to subtotal ablation thereby theoretically decreasing morbidity [25]. Several factors must be considered before focal therapy can be implemented as a routine option for early-stage prostate cancer. First, prostate cancer is often a multifocal disease. However, large studies have shown that between 10% and 44% of radical prostatectomy (RP) specimens harbor unilateral or unifocal cancers [26]. There is growing evidence that the majority of progression is driven by the size (>0.5 mL) and grade (Gleason ≥7) of the index tumor [27], and that most multifocal tumors outside the index lesion have a volume of <0.5 mL, making their clinical significance questionable. Some have argued that tumors <0.5 mL may not need immediate treatment [28], thus creating a large population of patients that may benefit from focal ablation of the index or unifocal tumor with subsequent surveillance of the smaller "clinically insignificant" lesions if present. (Figures 1.1a–h).

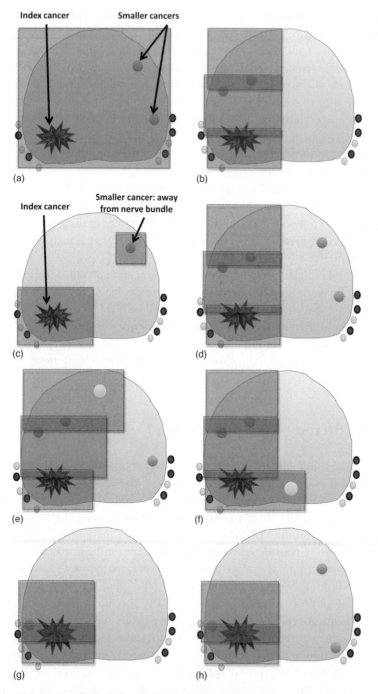

Figure 1.1 (a) Standard whole-gland strategies treat the entire prostate regardless of the risk category, volume, or disposition of cancer. (b–h) These figures illustrate the different strategies that could be employed using focal therapy to ablate either all areas of cancer or just the index lesion.

If focal therapy is to be considered, accurate localization of the index tumor is critical. Both improved biopsy as well as imaging techniques may allow for clearer and more accurate localization. Small prostate cancers have in the past proven to be very difficult to accurately detect radiographically, forcing most clinicians to rely on prostate biopsy to derive location and volume information. This trend is rapidly changing with improved imaging [29] and biopsy techniques such as transperineal template prostate mapping [30]. Given that benign PSA-producing tissue is spared with focal therapy, what constitutes appropriate cancer control measures (other than mortality) to be used in clinical trials is yet to be established. Composite definitions incorporating biochemical, histological, and imaging outcomes are likely to be needed until mature datasets demonstrate whether efficacy is maintained with respect to metastases and mortality [31].

Conclusion

Due to widespread screening, many contemporary prostate malignancies are small and focal in nature. Given the stage and tumor volume migration that has occurred, functional as well as cancer-specific outcomes are being critically assessed. Evidence is growing that novel techniques may offer similar disease control as the current "gold standards" while the treatment morbidity may be considerably less. Refinement and long-term assessment of the techniques described are critical if we are to better understand the role of such therapy in the management of prostate cancer.

References

1. Sandra MG, et al. Quality of life and satisfaction with outcome among prostate-cancer survivors. *NEJM* 2008;358: 1250.
2. Hu JC, et al. Comparative effectiveness of minimally invasive vs open radical prostatectomy. *JAMA* 2009;302(14): 1557–1564.
3. Cooperberg MR, Broering JM, Carroll PR. Time trends and local variation in primary treatment of localized prostate cancer. *JCO* 2010;28(7): 1117.
4. Kamangar F, et al. Patterns of cancer incidence, mortality, and prevalence across five continents: defining priorities to reduce cancer disparities in different geographic regions of the world. *JCO* 2006;24: 2137.
5. Konety BR, et al. Comparison of the incidence of latent prostate cancer detected at autopsy before and after the prostate specific antigen era. *J Urol* 2005;174: 1785.
6. Schröder FH, et al. ERSPC Investigators. Screening and prostate-cancer mortality in a randomized European study. *NEJM* 2009;360(13): 1320–1328.
7. Andriole GL, et al. PLCO Project Team. Mortality results from a randomized prostate-cancer screening trial. *NEJM* 2009;360(13): 1310–1319.

8. Zeliadt SB, et al. Trends in treatment costs for localized prostate cancer: the healthy screenee effect. *Med Care* 2007;45: 154.

9. Benoit RM, et al. Comparison of the hospital costs for radical prostatectomy and cryosurgical ablation of the prostate. *Urology* 1998;52(5): 820.

10. Greenberg D, et al. When is cancer care cost effective? *JNCI* 2010;102(2): 82–88.

11. Zietman A. Evidence-based medicine, conscience-based medicine, and the management of low-risk prostate cancer. *JCO* 2009;27(30): 4935–4936.

12. Chodak GW, et al. Results of conservative management of clinically localized prostate cancer. *NEJM* 1994;330(4): 242.

13. Lu-Yao GL, et al. Outcomes of localized prostate cancer following conservative treatment. *JAMA* 2009; 302: 1202.

14. Johansson JE, et al. Natural history of early, localized prostate cancer. *JAMA* 2004;291: 2713.

15. Bill-Axelson A, et al. Scandinavian Prostate Cancer Group Study Number 4. Radical prostatectomy versus watchful waiting in localized prostate cancer: the Scandinavian prostate cancer group-4 randomized trial. *JNCI* 2008;100(16): 1144–1154.

16. Klotz L. Active surveillance for prostate cancer: for whom? *JCO* 2005;23: 8165.

17. Dall'Era MA, et al. Active surveillance for the management of prostate cancer in a contemporary cohort. *Cancer* 2008; 112(12): 2664.

18. Donnelly BJ, et al. A randomized trial of external beam radiotherapy versus cryoablation in patients with localized prostate cancer. *Cancer* 2010;116(2): 323–330.

19. Katz A, Rewcastle JC. The current and potential role of cryoablation as a primary treatment for prostate cancer. Current reports. *Oncol Rep* 2003;5: 231.

20. Wilt TJ, et al. Systematic review: Comparative effectiveness and harms of treatments for clinically localized prostate cancer. *Ann Intern Med* 2008;148: 435.

21. Warmuth M, et al. Systematic review of the efficacy and safety of high-intensity focussed ultrasound for the primary and salvage treatment of prostate cancer. *Eur Urol* 2010;58(6): 803–815.

22. Ahmed HU, et al. Minimally-invasive technologies in uro-oncology: the role of cryotherapy, HIFU and photodynamic therapy in whole gland and focal therapy of localised prostate cancer. *Surg Oncol* 2009; 18(3): 219–232.

23. Ahmed HU, et al. Will focal therapy become a standard of care for men with localized prostate cancer? *Nat Rev Clin Onc* 2007;4(11): 632–642.

24. Lazzeri M, Guazzoni G. Focal therapy meets prostate cancer. *Lancet* 2010;376(9746): 1036–1037.

25. Ward JF, Jones JS. Classification system: organ preserving treatment for prostate cancer. *Urology* 2010;75(6): 1258 1260.

26. Karavitakis M, et al. Tumor focality in prostate cancer: implications for focal therapy. *Nat Rev Clin Onc* 2011;8(1): 48–55.

27. Wise AM, et al. Morphologic and clinical significance of multiple prostate cancers in radical prostatectomy specimens. *Urology* 2002; 60: 264.

28. Ahmed HU. The index lesion and the origin of prostate cancer. *NEJM* 2009;361(17): 1704–1706.

29. Ahmed HU, et al. Is it time to consider a role for MRI before prostate biopsy? *Nat Rev Clin Oncol* 2009; 6(4): 197–206.

30. Onik G, Barzell W. Transperineal 3D mapping biopsy of the prostate: an essential tool in selecting patients for focal prostate cancer therapy. *Urol Oncol* 2008;26(5): 506–510.

31. Ahmed HU, Emberton M. Benchmarks for success in focal therapy of prostate cancer: cure or control? *World J Urol* 2010;28(5): 577–582.

CHAPTER 2

Factors That Affect Patients' Choice of Treatment

Deb Feldman-Stewart PhD[1,2] and Michael D. Brundage MSc FRCPC MD[1,2,3,4]

[1] Division of Cancer Care and Epidemiology, Cancer Research Institute, Queen's University, Kingston, ON, Canada
[2] Department of Oncology, Queen's University, Kingston, ON, Canada
[3] Department of Community Health and Epidemiology, Queen's University, Kingston, ON, Canada
[4] Cancer Centre of Southeastern Ontario, Kingston, ON, Canada

Introduction

Choosing a treatment for early-stage prostate cancer often presents a very complicated decision for men. There are many standard therapies available, including radical prostatectomy, external beam radiation, brachytherapy, and watchful waiting (instituting palliative treatment if required) or active surveillance (instituting radical treatment only if specific indications appear). The situation is further complicated by the poor quality of evidence around the relative efficacy and the relevant outcomes of each treatment option (Figure 2.1).

Factors influencing patient choice

In this chapter, we are referring to information "factors," the facts and opinions that may affect a patient's choice.

Side effects versus efficacy

Clinicians have an intuitive understanding that the chances of cure, balanced against the risks to bladder, bowel, and sexual function, are powerful factors influencing treatment choices of both patients and clinicians. In this chapter, we review this common medical paradigm of factors that relate to balancing potential benefit against potential harm, and highlight complexities related to this seemingly straight-forward consideration of

Focal Therapy in Prostate Cancer, First Edition. Edited by Hashim U Ahmed, Manit Arya, Peter Carroll and Mark Emberton.
© 2012 Blackwell Publishing Ltd. Published 2012 by Blackwell Publishing Ltd.

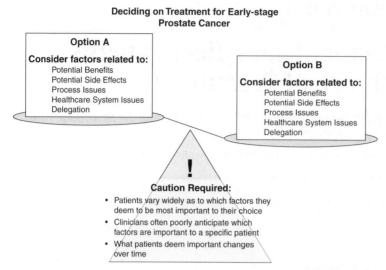

Figure 2.1 A diagram to illustrate how men choose between different therapies when diagnosed with localized prostate cancer.

competing outcomes. We then go on to show that this common paradigm (even acknowledging the complexities) is too limited in its approach to the decision, by identifying additional factors that patients often consider in making their choices.

Reviews of previous research on what factors influence patients choices in this decision agree that patients are motivated to have treatment to eradicate the cancer [1,2]. The reviews also report that patients do balance the potential benefit against possible harms, and consistent with clinicians' intuitive understanding, the treatment's potential impact on bladder, bowel functioning, and sexual functions is central to their discussion. However, in their review, Zeliadt et al. suggest that there appears to be a disconnect between what side effects patients say are important and what actually influences their decisions. The reviewers note that data on the issue come from different types of studies, including qualitative and quantitative, prospective and retrospective studies. Sorting out how data from these different studies fit together is a challenge, but it does reveal that the factors that affect men's treatment decisions are not just a simple list that is suggested earlier.

Underlying the complexities are three key themes: (1) there is high variability among patients in what affects their decisions; (2) detail matters—for example, particular details that affect the decision being unanticipated at times; and (3) the decision-making process is protracted in time. By piecing together qualitative and quantitative studies, we gain some insight into the extent of variability and into the importance of understanding and addressing details; by integrating prospective and retrospective studies, we gain some insight into longitudinal processes.

In the context of the common clinical paradigm, research addressing how the potential benefits of treatment influence choice illustrates all three complexity themes. An important longitudinal shift is that once men learn that efficacy does not differ greatly among the potential treatments, for many patients, it recedes as being a factor that affects the choice. However, variability is seen when looking at the details in a sensitivity assessment: an absolute difference, as small as 1%, in the chances of survival at 10 years would affect decisions of some men [3]. Another example in which the detail reveals high variability relates to cancer spread: some patients consider the chances that cancer will spread [4,5] to be important, while others consider *where* the cancer is likely to spread as most important. For example, potential brain metastases as opposed to other sites is a factor for some patients. A final detail around potential benefits reveals that some patients are concerned about whether there is a second-line treatment available should the first fail. Thus, factors related to potential benefit as suggested in the simple paradigm are not quite so simple.

Continuing with the common clinical paradigm, research on factors relating to patients' desire to avoid side effects also shows evidence of all three complexity themes. Variability can be seen in the fact that very few factors seem to affect the decisions of even half the patients; the most prevalent risk to avoid appears to be treatment's effect on bladder function [6,7]. Risk of impact on bowel and sexual functions has also been identified; each being the most important factor to some patients but not at all important to others. The variability is also evident in that, although a very rare side effect, the chance of treatment causing death is very important to some patients. The studies of detail show that many patients define their concerns in terms of the treatments' impact on their quality of life. This impact is articulated by some men as "impact on discomfort"; by others as impact on activities of daily life and by some as impact on their ability to work. For yet others, their concern is focussed more broadly to include all aspects of impact on their family and/or finances. Longitudinal effects are evident in factors relating to side effects, but rather than being systematic with respect to particular factors, as is seen with efficacy, they appear to be random. A large proportion of patients appear to demonstrate shifts in the factors that affect their decisions over time. This will be discussed later in the chapter.

Summarizing the above findings, many men seem to make this treatment decision by weighing factors considering cancer control against those considering side effects, the simple paradigm and a representation typified by decision analytic trees representing this decision [8]. The high variability among patients, the particular details that are important, and the shifts over time make the simple weighing of three primary potential side effects against one benefit an inadequate capture of what affects patients' decisions. Beyond this type of potential benefit versus side effect weighing, evidence suggests that many patients weigh other types of factors also. We have grouped these factors into three additional categories.

Process, healthcare system, and delegation

The first additional category of factors can be conceptualized as "process issues" around having the various treatments such as traveling required to get to treatment, being able to get a second opinion, how to know if the treatment was effective, how soon the treatment can start, the total length of time required for the treatment and time to recover. Other process issues relate to the procedures of the treatment itself, such as excision of the tumor (sometimes a pro, sometimes a con) or how to alleviate particular side effects [9].

A second additional category relates to the competency of the healthcare system. These factors include experience of the doctor, the experience of the nonphysician staff, the location where the treatment would be provided, and whether the equipment is up to date.

A final additional category of factors relates to the fact that the treatment decision is complicated, driving some patients to want assistance with the decision process or to delegate the decision to a trusted individual. For example, some patients seek the preferences of those who they view as more expert: the opinion of their doctors and also of other patients. Alternatively, some men use anecdotes of others' experiences, often without being clear about whether it is appropriate to generalize from these anecdotal situations.

Complex interaction of factors influencing decision-making

We have provided a rather extensive list of factors, and as noted previously, it appears that almost none of these are prevalent enough to affect the decision of more than half of the men choosing treatments for localized prostate cancer. It is worth asking if the apparent variability is due to the design of the studies that identified the factors. For example, inappropriate variability could arise because some studies include prostate cancer patients who do not have localized disease. Another cause of "inflated" variability relates to studies in which patients identify the important factors retrospectively, because the information actually provided to them beforehand limits what they can consider important. That information likely varies considerably across doctors since treatment patterns show high geographic variation in care, and evidence suggests that the information provided to patients is often slanted toward the physician's preference [10].

Valid estimates of variability can come from studies that ensure some baseline consistency in the information provided, such as studies of decision aids. We have created one such decision aid and designed it so that we can study aspects of the patients' cognitive processes while they happen, including identifying the factors that affect their decisions over the course of the decision. Under controlled circumstances, we found 33 different factors affected the decisions of 60 men, and each of 18 different factors was someone's "most important" factor. In that group, only two factor affected the decisions of 50% or more of patients: (1) the impact of the treatment on their bladder function the more prevalent; (2) and effect on bowel function the other. These data corroborate the impression of high variability suggested across the various studies reviewed and, as noted previously, were obtained after an explicit disclosure that PSA control was likely comparable with each treatment option discussed in the aid so that this did not factor heavily.

The decision-making process is protracted in time because, for many of these patients, this decision is "incomparable with any other life decisions" they had faced previously, in terms of complexity, seriousness, or both. New decisions demand particular cognitive processes, and understanding the processes can help clarify why the decision takes time and why important factors can change. With new information, patients can change their attitudes, as their understanding of the options improves and as they clarify their values. That is, in new decisions, people often need to discover which of their values are relevant and can discover that they have values that are in conflict with one another. For example, the values for quantity and also for quality of life. We noted previously that there is evidence of many shifts in the factors that affect patients' decisions over the time they make this decision, and in our decision aid study, 82% of our 60 patients changed either the factors they thought were important to selecting their most preferred option or the factors' relative impact (all had previously discussed their diagnosis and treatment options with both a urologist and a radiation oncologist). Thus, each study that looks at factors affecting decisions at just one point in time is only getting one snapshot in a process that can be quite extended and include many shifts.

Each of the complexities we have identified has implications both for clinicians and researchers. The high variability means that to cover the needs of the individual patient, either all patients need to receive all information—which risks overwhelming them—or information provision needs to be tailored to the needs of the individual. We note that efforts at identifying correlates of particular choices have not proved to be very helpful, since characteristics that have been statistically significant have been, at best, weak and, therefore, not useful for prediction [11]. We recognize that tailoring the information to individual patients is a clinical challenge and suggest that tools such as decision aids can help. The importance of particular details, some of which are unanticipated, increases the complexity of that challenge. The longitudinal nature of the decision processes further adds to that challenge, while it also highlights the disservice to patients who are not offered time to decide.

Conclusion

In summary, while patients are driven to choose treatment for early-stage prostate cancer by the desire to eradicate the cancer and limit unpleasant medical consequences, there are other important factors that influence many individuals. Factors related to the treatment processes, competency of the system, and those that help the decision-making process are examples of additional factors. Within each type of factor, the precise details that are important vary a great deal from one patient to another. In addition, the longitudinal nature of making this complex decision often results in a change of the factors that will ultimately affect the decision. Decision aids and structured provision of detailed information to men are recommended.

References

1. Zeliadt SB, et al. Why do men choose one treatment over another? A review of patient decision making for localized prostate cancer. *Cancer* 2006;106(9): 1865–1874.
2. Cox J, Amling CL. Current decision-making in prostate cancer therapy. *Cur Opin Urol* 2008;18: 275–278.
3. Brundage M, et al. Decision-making in early-stage prostate cancer: What factors are most relevant to patients? *Clin Inv Med* 2000;23(4 Supp): S19.
4. Feldman-Stewart D, et al. Patient-focussed decision-making in early-stage prostate cancer: Insights from a cognitively based decision aid. *Health Expectations* 2004;7: 126–141.
5. Feldman-Stewart D, et al. The information required by patients with early-stage prostate cancer in choosing their treatment. *BJU Int* 2001;87: 218–223.
6. Feldman-Stewart D, et al. The information needed by Canadian early-stage prostate cancer patients for decision-making: Stable over a decade. *Pat Ed Coun* 2008;73: 437–442.
7. Steginga S, et al. Making decisions about treatment for localized prostate cancer. *BJU Int* 2002;89: 255–260.
8. Walsh PC. A decision analysis of alternative treatment strategies for clinically localized prostate cancer. *J Urol* 1993;150: 1330–1332.
9. Denberg TD, et al. Patient treatment preferences in localized prostate carcinoma: the influence of emotion, misconception, and anecdote. 2006;107: 620–630.
10. Cohen H, Britten N. Who decides about prostate cancer treatment? A qualitative study. *Family Practice* 2003;20: 724–729.
11. Block CA, et al. Personality, treatment choice and satisfaction in patients with localized prostate cancer. *Int J Urol* 2007;14: 1013–1018.

CHAPTER 3

Histological Trends and the Index Lesion in Localized Prostate Cancer

Vladimir Mouraviev MD[1], Thomas M. Wheeler MD[2], and Thomas J. Polascik MD FACS[1,3,4]

[1] Division of Urology, Department of Surgery, University of Cincinnati College of Medicine, Cincinnati, OH
[2] Department of Pathology and Immunology, Baylor College of Medicine, Houston, TX, USA
[3] Division of Urologic Surgery and Duke Prostate Center (DPC), Department of Surgery, Duke University Medical Center, Durham, NC, USA
[4] Duke Cancer Institute, Duke University Medical Center, Durham, NC, USA

Introduction

Prostate cancer is a heterogeneous disease that may contain single or, more commonly, multiple tumor foci within the same gland. Various studies have reported that the majority of radical prostatectomy (RP) specimens (67–87%) contain multifocal disease [1]. Nonetheless, there is often an index tumor—as determined by the largest tumor volume and/or highest Gleason grade that is presumed to be the driver of prognosis—and one or more separate secondary tumors. Due to improvements in screening and prostate cancer detection, some men now present with early stage cancer that may be amenable to organ-sparing procedures, similar to the evolution of almost all other solid organ malignancies [2].

Multifocal, unifocal, and unilateral prostate cancer

The traditional approach to prostate cancer treatment is predicated upon tumor multifocality and heterogeneity, providing the foundation for radical whole-gland treatment using surgery, radiation, or minimally invasive thermoablative techniques. The multifocal nature of prostate cancer coupled to our inability to reliably detect such disease has to date maintained the status quo and hampered efforts to select appropriate candidates

Focal Therapy in Prostate Cancer, First Edition. Edited by Hashim U Ahmed, Manit Arya, Peter Carroll and Mark Emberton.
© 2012 Blackwell Publishing Ltd. Published 2012 by Blackwell Publishing Ltd.

for focal therapy. However, with the widespread introduction of prostate-specific antigen (PSA) screening and early detection of prostate cancer, many authors have reported an increased proportion of unifocal and unilateral disease. These are summarized in Table 3.1. Several studies suggest that 20–30% of men with low-risk disease may be candidates for tissue-preserving treatment approaches. As a result, and combined with the inability to accurately localize cancer foci, this has led most focal therapists to adopt the strategy of hemiablation of unilateral cancer as a reasonable compromise between the challenges of focal ablation of the tumor alone and the morbidity of whole-gland therapy [24].

The concept of prostate hemiablation has been developed to treat one-half of the prostate, including the index lesion and any other focus that happens to fall within that lobe. Mouraviev et al. [25] analyzed 1186 RP specimens identifying completely unilateral cancers in 227 (19%). The majority of unilateral tumors (72%) were low volume with a percent tumor involvement of ≤5%. These data also demonstrated a reasonably high rate of clinically significant (Gleason score ≥7) tumors among small-volume, unilateral prostate cancer. Another group found that the majority of small-volume prostate cancers are multifocal, often involving both sides of the prostate [5]. Tumors are located predominantly in the peripheral zone (79%) and the posterior aspect (84%) of the prostate. Of these small-volume cancers, 16% had high Gleason grades that were clinically significant [5]. A recent analysis of 1000 RP specimens from early stage prostate cancer patients was recently conducted [6]. The authors revealed that 18% of lesions were unilateral. If extracapsular extension were present, it was associated with the largest focus of cancer of all intraprostatic tumors. Therefore, the clinical implication of this data is that effective ablation of the index lesion may eradicate the tumor burden that clinically leads to locally invasive disease and possibly metastatic disease.

One study conducted in 538 patients with biopsy-proven unilateral disease identified clinically significant prostate cancer contralateral to a unilateral positive prostate biopsy in RP specimens of men with low- to moderate-risk disease [23]. Tumors contralateral to the positive biopsy side had adverse pathologic features in 24%; of these 15% had extraprostatic extension, 8% had percent tumor involvement >15%, 5% had Gleason score >7, 3% had seminal vesicle invasion, and the remaining 69% had a combination of these features. Another group retrospectively evaluated what could be missed on the contralateral side assuming a hemiablation procedure was performed for preoperatively identified unilateral disease by conventional, office-based prostate biopsy validated by final RP specimens in 100 cases [19]. They found that needle biopsy features of limited disease—less than three positive cores that were all unilateral, ≤50% involvement of any positive core, Gleason score ≤6—predicted unilateral clinically significant cancer accurately. In other words, from 66 cases only

Table 3.1 Unifocality and unilaterality on the basis of final pathological assessment of prostatectomy specimens.

	Study/group	Number of RP specimens	Risk category or tumor features of analyzed cohort	Processing method	%
Unifocality	Bastacky et al. [3] (Johns Hopkins)	27 sporadic 26 familial	All	3-mm sections	30 24
	Arora et al. [4] (Indiana)	115	All	Whole mount	13
	Cheng et al. [5] (Indiana)	62	TV < 0.5 cc	Whole mount	31
	Ohori et al. [6] (MSKCC/Baylor)	1000	Low-risk	Whole mount	18
	Villers et al. [7] (Stanford)	234	All	3-mm sections	50
	Wise et al. [8] (Stanford)	486	All	3-mm sections	17
	Noguchi et al. [9] (Stanford)	222	All	3-mm sections	24
	Rukstalis et al. [10] (MCP Heneman)	112	All	Whole mount	21
	Boccon-Gibod et al. [11] (Paris)	56	All	3-mm sections	30
	Djavan et al. [12] (Vienna)	308	All	4-mm sections	33
	Horninger et al. [13] (Innsbruck)	80	PSA ≤ 3.25 ng/mL	Whole mount	35
	Stamatiou K et al. [14] (Tzaneion, Greece)	40	Impalpable (cT1a)	4-mm sections	40
	Miller et al. [15] (Colorado)	151	All	Whole mount	44
	Song et al. [16] (Seoul)	132	All	Whole mount	67
	Karavitakis et al. [17] (London)	100	All	Whole mount	22
Unilaterality	Mouraviev et al. [18] (Duke*)	1184	Low-risk	3-mm sections	19
	Yoon et al. [19] (Johns Hopkins)	100	Low-risk	3-mm sections	31
	Cheng et al. [5] (Indiana)	62	TV < 0.5 cc	Whole mount	63
	Iczkowski et al. [21] (Colorado & Houston)	393	All	Whole mount	23
	Haffner et al. [22] (Lille)	106	All	Whole mount	28 PZ 11 TZ/AFMS
	Tareen et al. [23] (NYU)	1458	All	3–5-mm sections	21.3

TV, tumor volume; PZ, peripheral zone; TZ, transition zone; AFMS, anterior fibromuscular stroma.

one prostate cancer focus was identified in the contralateral lobe. In 65 RP specimens, there was tumor contralateral to the positive biopsy with a mean total tumor volume of 0.2 mL, one threshold for clinical significance that is widely adopted by many. However, clinically significant cancer according to the Epstein definition would have been missed in 20% of cases in the contralateral lobe if hemiablation were performed based on diagnostic biopsy [19]. This study further identifies the limited accuracy of conventional, office-based TRUS-guided prostate biopsy to select patients for hemiablation. Other authors have reported similar data that demonstrate that standard 6–12 core biopsy is not sufficient to rule out cancer in the contralateral lobe. Therefore, further progress to develop a more accurate tool for early stage prostate cancer detection in the contralateral lobe using optimal extended prostate biopsy is required. The optimal strategy is template prostate mapping. Image-guided techniques are ultimately required when selecting men for focal therapy.

One suggestion is that subtotal prostate parenchyma-sparing cryoablation—in which most of the gland is ablated except a small amount near the neurovascular bundles—may improve genitourinary outcomes without requiring increasing refinements in biopsy or imaging techniques. In a recent study, it was shown that cancer control could be accomplished with a 21% risk of significant (i.e., >0.5 mL) residual disease in which it was assumed that the largest tumor would be the one detected by biopsy, and the ablative area was restricted to 9 of 12 prostate zones [10]. In other words, the entire ipsilateral, peripheral, and transition zones, as well as contralateral peripheral zone (hockey-stick ablation), thereby sparing the contralateral neurovascular bundle [10]. Ward et al. also evaluated a possible efficacy of regional ablation on the basis of a retrospective analysis of 180 RP specimens with a unilateral positive prostate biopsy [26]. Most out-of-field cancers remained as clinically insignificant tumors and were not identified by prostate biopsy (low volume, 0.5 mL with low-grade Gleason score ≤6). The subtotal (hockey-stick template) encompassed all index tumors.

The index tumor

It has been argued that secondary small-volume tumors do not significantly influence the survival of patients after potentially completely eradicating the clinically significant index lesion(s) [27]. Pivotal work carried out by group from Stanford University [7,8] showed that pathologic evaluation of the index tumor accurately predicted the clinical behavior of the entire gland regardless of synchronous tumors in >90% of patients. Furthermore, they demonstrated that 80% of secondary

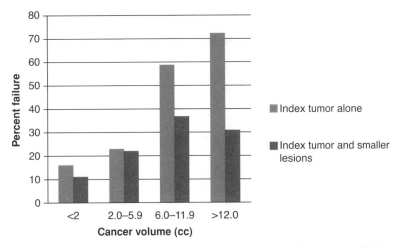

Figure 3.1 Clinical significance of index lesion versus multifocal lesions. (Modified from [8].)

tumors are <0.5 mL in the aggregate volume, another common criterion for depiction of clinical insignificance. When they searched for biological significance of small, independent cancers compared with the index tumor and its impact on biochemical disease-free survival, the Stanford group found that the biochemical disease-free survival rates were similar when considering only the index tumor volume compared to the index plus smaller tumor volume [8] (Figure 3.1).

In a study of 947 RP specimens between 1983 and 1998 to map and measure all tumor foci (Figure 3.2), a total of 389 cases had preoperative needle

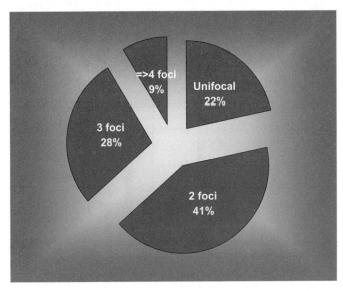

Figure 3.2 Distribution of unifocal and multifocal tumors.

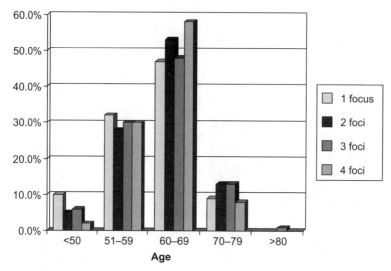

Figure 3.3 Age distribution in unifocal and multifocal tumors.

biopsy information available [24]. In summary, multifocality did not seem to depend on patient age ($p = 0.10$) (Figure 3.3) and multifocal tumors were more frequent (81%) in more recently diagnosed patients (Figure 3.4) [24]. In multivariate analysis the following factors significanctly contributed to multifocality: recent year of surgery ($p < 0.001$), higher clinical stage ($p = 0.002$), extracapsular extension ($p = 0.03$), seminal vesicle invasion ($p = 0.001$), and higher biopsy Gleason scores ($p = 0.04$). Other variables did not have an influence on multifocality, including preoperative PSA ($p = 0.43$), surgical margin status ($p = 0.86$), and lymph node status

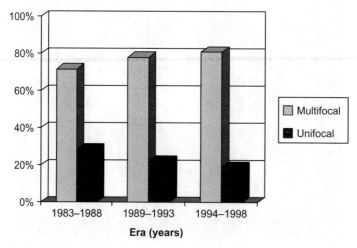

Figure 3.4 Change in multifocality by time period.

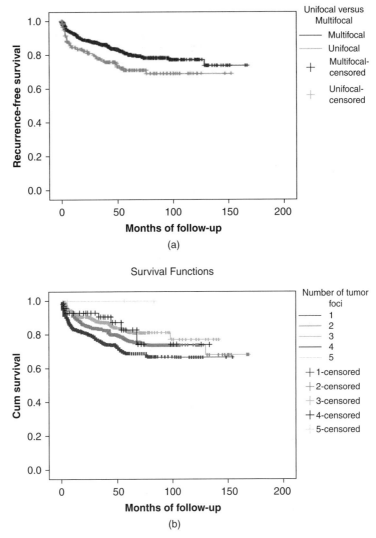

Figure 3.5 (a) Recurrence-free survival in unifocal versus multifocal tumors ($p = 0.043$). (b) Recurrence-free survival in tumors with different number of tumor foci ($p > 0.05$).

($p = 0.17$) [24]. Univariate Kaplan–Meier analysis demonstrated better biochemical-free survival for multifocal tumors versus a unifocal tumor ($p = 0.04$), although there were no significant differences between curves with the number of tumor foci ranging from 1 to 4 ($p > 0.05$) (Figure 3.5) [24]. Data from a larger cohort of 1184 RP specimens did not demonstrate a difference in biochemical outcomes between unilateral and bilateral tumors (Figure 3.6) [25]. From a tumor biology viewpoint, these data suggest that unilateral cancers represent a similar risk of PSA progression.

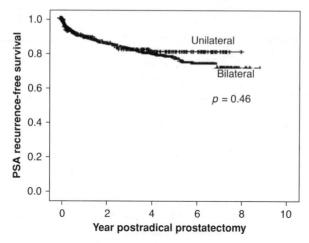

Figure 3.6 Kaplan–Meier PSA recurrence-free survival plot for unilateral and bilateral cancers.

Noguchi et al. [9] evaluated the prognostic value of small secondary cancers in multifocal, localized prostate cancer in a study of 222 men with T1c disease treated with RP. The cohort was divided into three groups, including (a) unifocal (24%), (b) index lesion with secondary lesions of total volume ≤0.5 mL (39%), and (c) index tumor with secondary cancers ≥0.5 mL (37%). The authors did not find a difference among the three groups with respect to preoperative PSA, number of positive cores, percent of Gleason pattern 4/5 (needle biopsy), or other histological features in RP specimens using multivariate analysis. Paradoxically, when comparing PSA failure rates among the three groups, the multifocal group with smaller secondary cancers had a better prognosis than the group with unifocal disease.

In a series of 100 whole-mount RP specimens, Karavitakis et al. [17] revealed 79% of all tumors as multifocal. However, even in multifocal disease, total tumor volume, Gleason Score, extracapsular extension, and seminal vesicle invasion were invariably defined by the index lesion. Of 170 satellite lesions, 147 (86%) had a total volume <0.5 mL and 169 (99%) had a Gleason score <6. In summary, although multiple prostate cancer foci are common, histopathological features of poor prognosis are correlated with the index lesion. In addition, about half the cases may have been suitable for index lesion ablation with surveillance of the remaining small low-grade satellite cancer lesions. Contrary to the preceding studies, Ruijter et al. [28] found that a quarter of the tumors invading the capsule in multifocal disease were not the index lesion, and that tumors need not acquire large volumes before they become locally invasive. Even foci as small as 0.2 mL in size may show a significant release of tumor cells into the blood stream and can give rise to lymph node metastasis [29]. In a series of 239 patients with tumor volume less than 0.5 mL, Kikuchi et al. [30] found that 43 were poorly differentiated, 11 had extracapsular extension, 6 had positive surgical margins, 2 had positive lymph nodes, and 7 experienced progression within 5 years.

Genetic studies on clonal origin of prostate cancer

Multifocality can be explained by either monoclonal or multiclonal expansion of tumor cells. The monoclonal hypothesis expounds that a single transforming event occurs in one cell with the spread of this clone through the organ resulting in topographically distinct but genetically related tumors. In other words, multifocality results from the intraprostatic metastasis of tumor cells. The multiclonal hypothesis suggests that an organ is under a field effect or propensity to develop tumors elsewhere and multiple tumors are, therefore, genetically distinct [31].

One way to investigate tumor clonality is to perform molecular analysis of microsatellite alterations. If prostate cancer is a single-clone disease, similar genetic alterations would be expected among different tumor foci within the same gland. Cheng et al. [32] studied the pattern of allelic losses on chromosomes 8p12-21 and in the *BRCA1* locus on chromosome 17q21. These genetic abnormalities have been associated with development and progression of prostate cancer. In most cases of distinctly separate tumors there was a random, discordant pattern of allelic loss, whereas the same pattern of allelic loss was noticed in DNA samples derived from different regions of the same tumor. These data suggest multiple prostate cancers arise independently and are probably secondary to numerous independent mutations rather than proliferation and intraglandular spread of a single malignant transformed cell.

However, monoclonality cannot be fully excluded. In a study of 25 different loci on 9 chromosomal arms for loss of heterozygosity, it was found that there is at least some degree of clonality in prostate cancer. Indeed, one could not rule out the possibility that separate tumors result from intraglandular dissemination, at least in some patients. Different patterns of allelic loss among multifocal tumors may simply be the result of clonal divergence after intraluminal spread rather than true oligoclonality. It is possible that at least in some cases, both field effect and monoclonal tumor expansion and intraglandular metastasis may coexist in the same patient.

It has been demonstrated that multiple tumors in the same prostate were genetically different; the chromosomal anomaly seen in lymph node metastases corresponded to that of the nondominant lesions in four cases concluding that the size and grade of the primary tumor focus were unreliable in predicting metastatic behavior. However, the secondary tumor, which was supposedly distinct from the index lesion, was in many cases very close to the larger lesion and could be regarded as part of the larger lesion [28]. A recent report from an international multicenter trial demonstrated a monoclonal origin of lethal prostate cancer [33]. The PELICAN (Project to Eliminate Lethal Prostate Cancer) study was started in 1994, whereby patients were consented to a postmortem autopsy assessing metastatic sites in those who died because of prostate cancer. The authors collected specimens of 94 anatomically separate cancer sites in 30 men evaluating the data using high-resolution genome-wide single nucleotide polymorphism and copy number surveys. The investigators demonstrated that lethal, metastatic prostate cancer maintained a unique genetic signature copy number pattern. In studying the role of TMPRSS2-ETS in tumor progression, it has equally been suggested that in spite of common genetic heterogeneity in primary prostate cancer, most metastatic cancers arise from a single precursor cancer cell [34]. If the life-threatening lesion can be identified and targeted at the very beginning of carcinogenesis, it would be reasonable to ablate it using a focal approach [35].

Conclusion

Localized prostate cancer is increasingly low volume and low grade with a significant proportion of unifocal and unilateral cancer. While the detection of a unifocal lesion remains challenging for early stage disease, patients with unilateral lesions may be reasonable candidates for hemiablation. Furthermore, clinically significant lesions (whether the index lesion or not) can be considered a driving force of prostate cancer progression and therefore should be ablated at an early stage. In general, satellite lesions do not appear to be life-threatening to the patient at the time that the index tumor is detected.

References

1. Mouraviev V, et al. Pathologic basis of focal therapy for early-stage prostate cancer. *Nat Rev Urol* 2009;6(4): 205–215.
2. Ahmed HU, et al. Will focal therapy become a standard of care for men with localized prostate cancer? *Nat Clin Pract Oncol* 2007;4(11): 632–642.
3. Bastacky SI, et al. Pathological features of hereditary prostate cancer. *J Urol* 1995;153: 987–992.
4. Arora R, et al. Heterogeneity of Gleason grade in multifocal adenocarcinoma of the prostate. *Cancer* 2004;100: 2362–2366.

5. Cheng L, et al. Anatomic distribution and pathologic characterization of small-volume prostate cancer (<0.5 ml) in whole-mount prostatectomy specimens. *Mod Pathol* 2005;18: 1022–1026.

6. Ohori M, et al. Is focal therapy reasonable in patients with early stage prostate cancer (CAP) – an analysis of radical prostatectomy (RP) specimens. *J Urol* 2006;175(Suppl) 507 (abstract 1574).

7. Villers A, et al. Multiple cancers in the prostate. Morphologic features of clinically recognized vs. incidental tumors. *Cancer* 1992;70: 2312–2318.

8. Wise AM, et al. Morphologic and clinical significance of multifocal prostate cancers in radical prostatectomy specimens. *Urology* 2002;60(2): 264–269.

9. Noguchi M, et al. Prognostic factors for multifocal prostate cancer in radical prostatectomy specimens: lack of significance of secondary cancers. *J Urol* 2003;170 (2 Pt 1): 459–463.

10. Rukstalis DB, et al. Prostate cryoablation: a scientific rationale for future modifications. *Urology* 2002;60(2 Suppl 1): 19–25.

11. Boccon-Gibod LM, et al. Micro-focal prostate cancer: a comparison of biopsy and radical prostatectomy specimen features. *Eur Urol* 2005;48: 895–899.

12. Djavan B, et al. Predictability and significance of multifocal prostate cancer in the radical prostatectomy specimen. *Tech Urol* 1999;5: 139–142.

13. Horninger W, et al. Characteristics of prostate cancers detected at low PSA levels. *Prostate* 2004;58(3): 232–237.

14. Stamatiou K, et al. Frequency of impalpable prostate adenocarcinoma and precancerous conditions in Greek male population: an autopsy study. *Prostate Cancer Prostatic Dis* 2006;9(1): 45–49.

15. Miller GJ, Cygan JM. Morphology of prostate cancer: the effects of multifocality on histological grade, tumor volume and capsule penetration. *J Urol* 1994;152(5) (Pt 2): 1709–1713.

16. Song SY, et al. Pathologic characteristics of prostatic adenocarcinomas: a mapping analysis of Korean patients. *Prostate Cancer Prostatic Dis* 2003;6: 143–147.

17. Karavitakis M, et al. Histological characteristics of the index lesion in whole-mount radical prostatectomy specimens: implications for focal therapy. *Prostate Cancer Prostatic Dis* 2011;14(1): 46–52.

18. Mouraviev V, et al. Prostate cancer laterality as a rationale of focal ablative therapy for the treatment of clinically localized prostate cancer. *Cancer* 2007;110(4): 906–910.

19. Yoon GS, et al. Residual tumor potentially left behind after local ablation therapy in prostate adenocarcinoma. *J Urol* 2008;179: 2203–2206.

20. Iczkowski KA, et al. *Urology* 2008;71(6): 1166–1171.

21. Haffner J, et al. Peripheral zone prostate cancers: location and intraprostatic patterns of spread at histopathology. *Prostate* 2009;69: 276–282.

22. Tareen B, et al. Laterality alone should not drive selection of candidates for hemi-ablative focal therapy. *J Urol* 2009;181: 1082–1089.

23. Polascik TJ, et al. Pathologic stage T2a and T2b prostate cancer in the recent prostate-specific antigen era: implications for unilateral ablative therapy. *Prostate* 2008;68(13): 1380–1386.

24. Wheller TM. Personal communication. 2009

25. Mouraviev V, et al. Prostate cancer laterality as a rationale of focal ablative therapy for the treatment of clinically localized prostate cancer. *Cancer* 2007;110(4): 906–910.

26. Ward JF, et al. Cancer ablation with regional templates applied to prostatectomy specimens from men who were eligible for focal therapy. *BJUInt* 2009;104(4): 490–497.

27. Karavitakis M, et al. Tumor focality in prostate cancer: implications for focal therapy. *Nat Rev Clin Oncol* 2011;8(1): 48–55.

28. Ruijter ET, et al. Molecular analysis of multifocal prostate cancer lesions. *J Pathol* 1999;188(3): 271–277.

29. Gburek BM, et al. Chromosomal anomalies in stage D1 prostate adenocarcinoma primary tumors and lymph node metastases detected by fluorescence in situ hybridization. *J Urol* 1997;157(1): 223–227.

30. Kikuchi E, et al. Is tumor volume an independent prognostic factor in clinically localized prostate cancer? *J Urol* 2004;172(2): 508–511.

31. Kallioniemi OP, Visakorpi T. Genetic basis and clonal evolution of human prostate cancer. *Adv Cancer Res* 1996;68: 225–255.

32. Cheng L, et al. Evidence of independent origin of multiple tumors from patients with prostate cancer. *JNCI* 1998;90(3): 233–237.

33. Liu W, et al. Copy number analysis indicates monoclonal origin of lethal metastatic prostate cancer. *Nat Med* 2009;15(5): 559–565.

34. Mehra R, et al. Characterization of TMPRSS2-ETS gene aberrations in androgen-independent metastatic prostate cancer. *Cancer Res* 2008;68(10): 3584–3590.

35. Ahmed HU. The index lesion and the origin of prostate cancer. *NEJM* 2009;361(17): 1704–1706.

CHAPTER 4

Selection Criteria for Prostate Cancer Focal Therapy

Rajat K. Jain[1], Timothy K. Ito[2], and Samir S. Taneja[2,3]

[1]New York University Langone Medical Center, School of Medicine, New York, NY, USA
[2]Division of Urologic Oncology, Department of Urology, New York University Langone Medical Center, New York, NY, USA
[3]Urology Section, Veterans Administration, New York Harbor Healthcare System (Manhattan campus), New York, NY, USA

Introduction

Focal therapy aims to selectively destroy a focus of prostate cancer while leaving normal prostate unharmed. Such a strategy relies heavily on the ability to identify disease location with great accuracy by either imaging or saturation biopsy techniques. As the accuracy of mapping declines, larger amounts of prostate must be destroyed in order to ensure efficacy. As such, criteria and methods for candidate selection in prostate cancer focal therapy might vary according to the amount of tissue to be destroyed, the intent or goal of therapy, and the risk category of the patient to be treated. In this chapter, we review the influence of treatment philosophy on candidate selection and the merits and limitations of current selection methodologies.

In order to distinguish methods of focal therapy delivery, we have developed a nomenclature at New York University (referred to in this chapter) allowing distinction of the goals of treatment: (1) lesion-ablative therapy (LAT), implying destruction of only a cancerous focus; (2) hemiablative therapy (HAT), destroying a whole-prostate lobe; or (3) subtotal ablative therapy (STAT), sparing only the posterolateral region of the uninvolved side (Figure 4.1). The method of delivery is heavily dependent upon the intent of therapy and the method of mapping.

Focal Therapy in Prostate Cancer, First Edition. Edited by Hashim U Ahmed, Manit Arya, Peter Carroll and Mark Emberton.

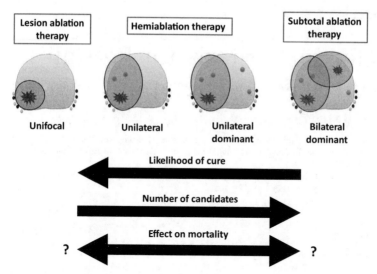

Figure 4.1   Cure versus control: influence of treatment goal on patient selection. As the number and distribution of cancerous foci increases, a larger and larger area of the prostate must be destroyed. This results in three modalities of focal therapy: lesion-ablative therapy (LAT), hemiablative therapy (HAT), and subtotal ablative therapy (STAT). The number of men qualifying for curative intent treatment depends on the amount of prostate the surgeon is willing to destroy. Most men with low-risk disease would become candidates for focal therapy as a method of disease control.

Goals of therapy

Curative intent

In its simplest form, focal therapy can be considered a curative therapy. In this form, the goal of therapy is complete eradication of disease through selective destruction of an area of the prostate. By extension then, candidate selection must be focused upon identification of men with low-risk, minimal volume disease confined to a specific area of the prostate. The number of men qualifying for such a treatment would vary, depending upon the amount of prostate targeted. In this application, focal therapy mimics radical therapy in its desired therapeutic outcome.

Disease control and prolongation of natural history

Focal therapy could be considered as a method of disease control, with the therapeutic intent being to prolong the natural history of disease, thereby avoiding or delaying radical therapy. This would place focal therapy as an adjunct to surveillance. By destroying the dominant focus of disease, or index lesion, with minimal toxicity, the surgeon secondarily prolongs the acceptable period of surveillance, perhaps minimizing the necessity for frequent biopsy, and allowing the patient relief from the anxiety of surveillance in the absence of definitive therapy. Utilizing this standard, most men with low-risk disease become candidates for focal therapy. Critical in this application is the ability to identify and map the site of dominant disease. While provocative, the ultimate influence on survival is unknown.

Noncurative intent and multimodal therapy

Finally, focal therapy could be considered as a component of a multimodal approach among high-risk patients. Given that single modality radical therapy is infrequently curative among men with high-risk disease, avoidance of the morbidity of radical therapy through use of alternate means of local control may be desirable. While this goal of focal therapy is perhaps most provocative, its implementation remains difficult in the absence of concept validation among low-risk candidates.

Who is the ideal candidate?

Low-risk or high-risk

A critical element in the selection of candidates is the decision of whether to limit focal therapy to men with low-risk disease. A clear advantage of doing so is minimization of the impact of treatment failure on survival, but a disadvantage is minimization of impact on survival in the case of treatment success. By including only low-risk candidates in early trials of focal therapy, it is likely that treatment failure would represent a failure of locoregional therapy, either due to inadequate mapping or ablation. Because early trials of focal therapy will likely be evaluated on the basis of local control rather than survival, it is perhaps imperative that systemic failure not *muddy the waters* as much as possible. A more difficult question then is how best to define low or acceptably low risk. In this regard, there is a great deal of controversy.

Prostate cancer has a varied natural course. Preoperative risk stratification provides prognostic information as well as a basis for treatment modality selection. The most commonly used definition of a clinically low-risk patient was published by D'Amico et al.: PSA <10 ng/mL and biopsy Gleason score <7 and clinical stage <T2b. Other numerous risk stratification nomograms are also used. Risk stratification can be used to assess likelihood of adverse pathology, poor oncological outcome, posttreatment biochemical recurrence, and ultimately survival. There is significant clinical evidence to suggest that patients categorized as low-risk harbor a very low likelihood of short-term cancer mortality.

Tareen et al. showed that in patients undergoing radical prostatectomy (RP), those classified as low-risk were significantly less likely to have positive margins, extracapsular extension (ECE) and pathologic Gleason score ≥7 [1]. Polascik et al. demonstrated that in a cohort of 538 low-risk patients, 81% had organ-confined disease, 92.7% of patients had pathological Gleason ≤7, and 70% had negative surgical margins [2]. D'Amico et al. similarly showed that in low-risk patients with a single microfocus of disease, only 6% had ECE, 79% had a pathologic Gleason score of ≤6, and 89% had negative surgical margins, while another study showed a 1% rate of ECE among low-risk patients [3].

While unifocal disease does appear to predict a low likelihood of adverse pathology, it is not clear that focality itself predicts risk. Tareen et al. reported that in a contemporary RP cohort, patients with unilateral disease were significantly more likely to have percent tumor involvement (PTI) ≤10%, organ-confined disease, and pathologic Gleason <7 [4]. However, further evaluation of the cohort demonstrated that while men with unilateral disease were more likely to have low-risk disease, those with bilateral low-risk disease fared similarly with regard to pathologic and oncologic outcome from prostatectomy. Similarly results have been noted by others, reporting favorable pathology among those with low-risk disease, and a 12% rate of biochemical recurrence for patients with unilateral disease and 14% for those with bilateral disease ($p = 0.25$) [5] .

Cure versus control: the concept of index lesion

Prostate cancer is a multifocal disease with only 13–38% of cases being truly unifocal (see Chapter 2). The prevalence of unilateral disease in contemporary RP cohorts is estimated at 21–23%. Curative intent therapy would limit the number of men qualifying for focal therapy to those with limited focality. Only 11% of the population currently undergoing RP has low-risk, unilateral disease. Identification of men with focally limited disease would require aggressive mapping strategies, making it difficult to widely implement. Furthermore, studies have shown that genetically heterogeneous cancerous foci arise independently of each other during the disease process. This genetic heterogeneity results in varying degrees of malignant potential, manifesting most commonly as one large dominant tumor focus (the "index lesion") complemented by smaller secondary lesions. Significant evidence exists that this index lesion drives the natural history of prostate cancer [6]. Studies also show that index tumor volume was equal to or greater than the total volume of all other tumor foci in 82% of RP specimens, and that the index lesion comprised a mean of 80% of the total tumor volume. Wise et al. demonstrated a mean and median ratio of secondary cancer volume to index cancer volume of 15% and 6%, respectively, with 96% of index cancers accounting for greater than half of the total cancer volume [7]. The index lesion volume has been shown to be independently predictive of PSA recurrence. A pathologic analysis of cystoprostatectomy specimens revealed that 80% of secondary cancers found incidentally were smaller than 0.5 mL in volume. A similar analysis of RP specimens showed that mean index lesion volume was 1.6 mL versus 0.3 mL for secondary lesions and that in 79% of patients, clinically significant cancer would be eradicated if the index disease were destroyed. The index lesion typically contains the highest grade disease, is more likely to be in concordance with the overall Gleason score, and to be the origin of adverse pathological features. The index lesion is the origin for ECE in 73–100% of cases. In one analysis, all cases of positive surgical margins and seminal vesicle invasion were associated with the index lesion. Meanwhile, another study showed that only 3% of secondary lesions contained high-grade components.

Methods of mapping

TRUS biopsy

Systematic transrectal ultrasound (TRUS)-guided prostate biopsy has emerged as the standard of care since being introduced in 1989. As most urologists are well trained and comfortable with techniques of TRUS biopsy, it is appealing to propose the technique for selection of candidates for focal therapy. Extended core and saturation biopsy techniques have increased cancer detection rates by 11–25% without increasing morbidity, but, nonetheless TRUS biopsy still has a high false negative rate. This observation leads one to suspect a substantial risk of understaging, undergrading, and missing disease foci.

Several authors have evaluated the ability of TRUS biopsy to predict final pathological characteristics. Divrik et al. suggest that the consensus from 20 well-designed studies is that concordance with pathological grade is highest when ≥10 cores are taken [8]. Studies show a Gleason score concordance of 70–76%, with 11–23% undergrading, and 6–10% overgrading. Grossklaus et al. found that in a multivariate analysis, increasing PSA, bilateral positive cores, and PTI were correlated with pathologic tumor volume and ECE [9]. Two similar analyses showed that PTI, PSA, and clinical Gleason score are correlated with tumor volume and risk of ECE. These data suggest that accurate pathologic correlation of biopsy data requires inclusion of additional clinical parameters.

Scales et al. recently undertook such a study evaluating 261 patients from the SEARCH database with T1c Gleason 6 disease and found only a 35% positive predictive value of a unilateral biopsy when compared to final RP pathologic specimen [10]. Tareen et al. found that among 590 men with unilateral cancer on biopsy, only 26% had true unilateral disease on final RP [11]. Upon further stratification to low-risk features, (PSA < 10 ng/mL, clinical stage T1c, Gleason <7) no clinical characteristic increased the accuracy of detecting unilateral cancer. Grossklaus et al. found no difference in the prediction of unilateral disease among men who had 6 or less biopsy cores with those who had greater than 6 cores. In the series of Tareen et al., positive predictive value for unilateral disease similarly did not improve for patients with 6, 6–12, or >12 cores. As such, use of TRUS biopsy for candidate selection may be limited to STAT applications or HAT in the setting of index lesion targeting.

Transperineal biopsy

Given the limitations of TRUS biopsy in mapping disease, many advocate a systematic, three-dimensional mapping technique taking samples every 5 mm using a brachytherapy-like templates [12] (see Chapter 5). In recent years, transperineal three-dimensional prostate mapping (TPM) biopsy has largely been used as a secondary tool in patients with previously negative TRUS biopsies. Studies evaluating a template biopsy strategy using fewer samples of 18–24 cores report a 23–47% cancer detection rate [13]. Several groups have used TPM to map the entire prostate, with 5 mm intervals between each core, demonstrating a 37–42% cancer detection rate [14, 15]. Several studies highlight the superiority of TPM to conventional biopsy techniques in restaging patients previously diagnosed with unilateral prostate cancer by TRUS biopsy; it has been demonstrated that 55–61% actually had bilateral cancer and 23% of patients had their Gleason score increased to 7 or higher. Overall, 69–76% had at least one finding on TPM that would have potentially changed their management. A similar study by Barzell and Melamed showed that of 80 patients with unilateral disease on TRUS biopsy, 54% had bilateral disease on TPM, and 16% had their Gleason score increased. Interestingly, when compared to TPM, repeat TRUS biopsy had a much higher false-negative rate and much lower relative sensitivity and specificity [16]. These results in combination indicate that, as a means of repeat biopsy, TPM is superior to repeat TRUS biopsy.

Imaging

Historically, imaging has added relatively little to prostate cancer mapping. Due to the invasive nature of transperineal biopsies, the use of imaging modalities to replace or improve current-mapping techniques is highly desirable, particularly in planning LAT. Several authors have investigated a multitude of modalities in this regard. Ultrasound techniques such as color and power Doppler generally lack the specificity necessary, and are quite operator dependent. Novel imaging techniques relying on radio-frequency feedback (Histoscanning®) offer potential for more accurate selection of abnormal regions of the prostate on ultrasound (see Chapter 6). Magnetic resonance imaging (MRI) currently provides the most accurate imaging modality for lesion detection and staging. Detection of cancerous foci has relied historically on T2-weighted (T2W) imaging that has been reported to have a widely varied sensitivity and specificity with regard to tumor localization (41–84%, 50–92%) and tumor staging (17–91%, 33–100%) (see Chapters 7, 8, and 9).

Recommendations

Selection of candidates for focal therapy is highly dependent upon the goal of therapy, the planned method of treatment, and the philosophy of the treating physician. Common to most treatment philosophies is the assertion that, for now, focal ablative therapies are best limited to men with low-risk disease. While improved mapping techniques may allow accurate selection of men with early localized intermediate or high-risk disease, at present inclusion of such men may risk early treatment failure, thereby rendering interpretation of therapeutic efficacy difficult. As such, inclusion of low-risk men, by conventional criteria, maximizes the likelihood of including men with organ-confined disease, and carries a low risk of early metastatic progression.

In selecting men for potentially curative focal therapy, demonstration of unifocal or unilateral disease for a planned LAT or HAT procedure is essential. Given the limitations of TRUS biopsy and imaging, at present transperineal template biopsy, typically using a 5-mm sampling frame, is a requirement of accurate candidate selection. If planning focal therapy as a means of altering the natural history of prostate cancer through destruction of the index lesion or dominant focus of disease, imaging may add greatly to candidate selection. Visible lesions are particularly well suited for LAT, and if MR-imaging strategies can adequately identify the index lesion they may represent the ideal means of candidate selection. While TPM biopsy remains the gold standard for identifying the index lesion, it is appealing to think that TRUS biopsy in combination with imaging may allow accurate identification in a less invasive fashion. Finally, if a STAT is planned, less aggressive biopsy strategies aimed at ruling out dominant disease may be employed. Ultimately, a strong desire in candidate selection will be to make it as noninvasive as feasible. Removing the need for repeat biopsy through modification of existing diagnostic biopsy templates is highly desirable and may become a reality through the integration of computerized biopsy templates and refinement of the goals of therapy.

References

1. Tareen B, et al. Laterality alone should not drive selection of candidates for hemi-ablative focal therapy. *J Urol* 2009;181(3): 1082–1090.
2. Polascik T, et al. Patient selection for hemiablative focal therapy of prostate cancer: variables predictive of tumor unilaterality based upon radical prostatectomy. *Cancer* 2009;115(10): 2104–10.
3. D'Amico AV, et al. Pathologic findings and prostate specific antigen outcome after radical prostatectomy for patients diagnosed on the basis of a single microscopic focus of prostate carcinoma with a gleason score </= 7. *Cancer* 2000;89(8): 1810–1817.
4. Tareen B, et al. Appropriate candidates for hemiablative focal therapy are infrequently encountered among men selected for radical prostatectomy in contemporary cohort. *Urology* 2009;73(2): 351–354.
5. Mouraviev V, et al. Prostate cancer laterality as a rationale of focal ablative therapy for the treatment of clinically localized prostate cancer. *Cancer* 2007;110(4): 906–910.
6. Ahmed HU. The index lesion and the origin of prostate cancer. *NEJM* 2009;361(17): 1704–1706.
7. Wise AM, et al. Morphologic and clinical significance of multifocal prostate cancers in radical prostatectomy specimens. *Urology* 2002;60(2): 264–269.
8. Divrik RT et al. Increasing the number of biopsies increases the concordance of Gleason scores of needle biopsies and prostatectomy specimens. *Urol Onc;* 25(5): 376–382.
9. Grossklaus DJ, et al. Percent of cancer in the biopsy set predicts pathological findings after prostatectomy. *J Urol* 2002;167(5): 2032–2036.
10. Scales CD, Jr et al. Predicting unilateral prostate cancer based on biopsy features: implications for focal ablative therapy–results from the SEARCH database. *J Urol* 2007;178(4Pt1): 1249–1252.
11. Tareen B, et al. Can contemporary transrectal prostate biopsy accurately select candidates for hemi-ablative focal therapy of prostate cancer? *BJUInt* 2009;104(2): 195–199.
12. Onik G, et al. Three-dimensional prostate mapping biopsy has a potentially significant impact on prostate cancer management. *JCO* 2009;27(26): 4321–4326.
13. Taira AV, et al. Performance of transperineal template-guided mapping biopsy in detecting prostate cancer in the initial and repeat biopsy setting. *Pros-Can-Pros-Dis* 2009.
14. Merrick GS, et al. Prostate cancer distribution in patients diagnosed by transperineal template-guided saturation biopsy. *Eur Urol* 2007;52(3): 715–724.
15. Li H, et al. Transperineal ultrasound-guided saturation biopsies using 11-region template of prostate: report of 303 cases. *Urology* 2007;70(6): 1157–1161.
16. Barzell W, Melamed M. Appropriate patient selection in the focal treatment of prostate cancer: the role of transperineal 3-dimensional pathologic mapping of the prostate—a 4-year experience. *Urology* 2007;70(6 Suppl): 27–35.

SECTION II

How can we accurately locate cancer within the gland?

CHAPTER 5

Localization of Cancer within the Gland: Biopsy Strategies

Winston E. Barzell MD FRCS FACS[1] and Rodrigo Pinochet MD[2,3]

[1]FSU College of Medicine, Urology Treatment Center, Sarasota, FL, USA
[2]Memorial Sloan-Kettering Cancer Center, New York, USA
[3]Department of Urology, Pontificia Universidad Catolica de Chile, Santiago, Chile

Introduction

A common conceptual criticism of focal therapy is that prostate cancer is often multifocal. Indeed patients with seemingly low-volume disease detected by office transrectal ultrasound biopsy (TRUS-biopsy) are frequently shown to have more advanced cancer on radical prostatectomy specimens in terms of stage, grade, and multifocality. Consequently, it is important that the selection process for patients undergoing focal therapy not include patients with clinically significant cancer outside the area destined to be ablated. Given this background, we will examine different prostate biopsy strategies and their role in the evaluation of patients for focal ablation.

Transrectal biopsy strategies

Transrectal systematic biopsies

Systematic sextant biopsies under transrectal ultrasound guidance (TRUS-biopsy) were introduced into clinical practice in 1989 by Hodge and remained the gold standard for several years. Because of the high false-negative rate of these sextant biopsies, extended biopsy protocols were introduced by many to maximize cancer detection rates. Eskew et al. described a 5-region technique incorporating lateral and midline biopsies with traditional sextant cores (total 13), which enhanced the detection rate to 40% [1]. The improved cancer detection rates using a 12-core biopsy strategy, which includes the classic sextant distribution with another set of sextant biopsies directed more laterally, provide the basis for the current wide use of this biopsy scheme.

Focal Therapy in Prostate Cancer, First Edition. Edited by Hashim U Ahmed, Manit Arya, Peter Carroll and Mark Emberton.
© 2012 Blackwell Publishing Ltd. Published 2012 by Blackwell Publishing Ltd.

Transrectal saturation biopsies

Others have proposed a technique of "saturation" biopsies to increase cancer detection and to better estimate the tumor extent and grade [2]. When saturation TRUS-biopsy is used as a repeat diagnostic procedure, the cancer detection rate is around 30–40% [3]. While saturation biopsies appear to detect more cancers than extended biopsies, the accuracy with which any TRUS-biopsy scheme can determine the size, location, extent, and grade of cancer remains to be demonstrated. In an effort to solve the latter shortcoming, a novel three-dimensional TRUS biopsy system, TargetScan® (Envisioneering Medical Technologies, St. Louis, Mo., USA) has been described recently. This system uses a three-dimensional imaging and targeting system to biopsy the prostate in a template fashion with flexible needles that can angle into the prostate. Preliminary studies reported a 47.6% cancer detection rate in patients with no previous biopsies. Furthermore, this approach appears superior to conventional TRUS-biopsy in terms of characterizing tumor size, location, and Gleason score [4].

Transperineal biopsy strategies

The efficacy of focal therapy remains unproven, and validated criteria for identifying patients who can safely be managed by this modality do not exist. Therefore, it is incumbent upon us to exclude patients who may unknowingly harbor more extensive significant cancer than predicted by the initial office TRUS-biopsy. In our opinion, this is currently best accomplished by proceeding with a comprehensive restaging procedure prior to selective ablation. Many physicians prefer a transperineal three-dimensional template-guided pathologic mapping (3D-TPM) approach for restaging [5,6], a perspective shared by Onik [7] and Crawford and Barqawi [8]. Advantages of the transperineal approach include: a ready access to the anterior apical areas of the prostate; a systematic approach to sampling that does not rely on visual three-dimensional recall and provides a fixed reproducible set of XYZ coordinates for use in cancer mapping, treatment planning, and follow-up; and a decreased likelihood of infection and bleeding. Furthermore, there are inherent difficulties in translating the findings from saturation TRUS-biopsy schemes to a Cartesian coordinate transperineal grid system through which most current ablative modalities used in focal therapy are delivered. The disadvantages of 3D-TPM are that it requires logistical support with specimen handling and labeling, is more costly, and requires either a general, regional, or local anesthesia.

The 3D-TPM-biopsy technique has been previously described (Figures 5.1 and 5.2). Biopsies with specific XYZ coordinates, may be individually labeled and submitted, or alternatively individual biopsies may be grouped

Prostate as seen by transrectal ultrasound during saturation biopsy

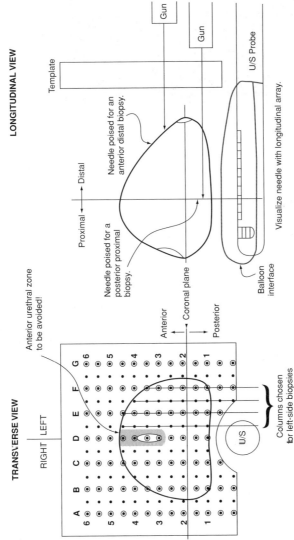

Figure 5.1 Prostate as seen by transrectal ultrasound during saturation biopsy. Please note that once a column is selected for biopsy, the needle should be manipulated so that its course can be visualized with the longitudinal array as illustrated. During this maneuver, it is crucial to maintain a fixed sagittal orientation of the ultrasound (U/S) probe. This technique prevents the needle from tracking and sampling outside the area intended for biopsy. While one is performing these biopsies, it is crucial to avoid injury to the prostatic urethra. This is accomplished by keeping a catheter in place to readily identify the urethra, and then by steering the biopsy needle away from this area. It is also important that midline biopsies are taken posterior to the urethra only because anterior midline biopsies will injure the urethra. (Reprinted with permission from Barzell WE, Whitmore WF III. Transperineal template guided saturation biopsy of the prostate: rationale, indications, and technique. *Urology Times* 2003;31:41–42.)

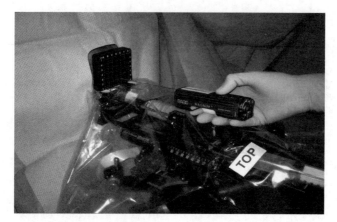

Figure 5.2   Operating room sterile setup.

together into zones (Figure 5.3), from which a pathologic map is generated (Figure 5.4). The University College London group has modified these template groups originally described by Barzell into "Modified
Barzell zones" (Figure 5.5). When considering focal therapy, and specifically hemigland ablation, it is important to segregate the midline biopsies
posterior to the urethra to prevent a "false positive" cancer reading from
the side destined to be untreated. Due to the "bevel" tracking, which is
a feature of most biopsy needles, a needle can inadvertently travel across
the midline from a location free of cancer and sample a cancerous region
on the opposite side. As this is a critical area for ablation because of its
proximity to the urethra and rectal wall, separating these midline biopsies
into a "neutral zone" is advisable.

Our initial practice was to leave an indwelling Foley catheter following
the procedure, but in the past 100 patients a post-op catheter has not been
routinely utilized. By meticulous avoidance of the urethral and bladder
mucosa in the biopsies, significant urinary bleeding should be an exceed-
ingly rare event. Complications with 3D-TPM are usually minor [9]. In our
study cited below, 12 of 140 patients (8.6%) developed minor complications (none requiring hospitalization), including urinary retention ($n = 6$),
worsening LUTS ($n = 2$) [2], and fever, scrotal edema, significant gross
hematuria, perineal ecchymosis ($n = 1$ each).

In an expansion of our initial retrospective study [5], we analyzed
the data on 140 patients who presented to one of the authors (Barzell)
between 2001 and 2009 with unilateral cancer deemed suitable for hemiablation based on an office TRUS-biopsy. These patients underwent a
restaging procedure that included 3D-TPM with a concomitant *repeat*
TRUS-biopsy. Patients were considered suitable for focal therapy if there
was no cancer on the side contralateral to the presenting lesion as noted on

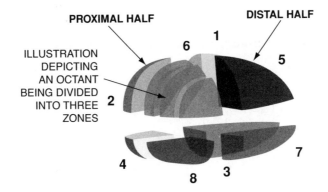

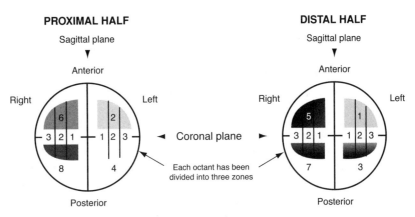

Figure 5.3 Specimen organization. The prostate is divided into proximal and distal halves, and each half is divided into four quadrants yielding eight octants. Each prostate octant is further divided into three zones, and the midline biopsies are segregated. Number of specimen jars = 24 zones + 2 midline (proximal/distal) + 2 to 8 TRUS (total = 28–34).

initial office TRUS-biopsy. Of the 140 patients, only 67 (48%) were suitable for FT using this strict definition, a finding consistent with reports by Onik et al. [7]. When comparing 3D-TPM to repeat TRUS-biopsy in determining suitability for focal treatment, 52% were found to be unsuitable by 3D-TPM while only 6.4% were deemed unsuitable by TRUS-biopsy. Additionally, repeat TRUS-biopsy had a false-negative rate of 52%, a sensitivity of 34%, and a negative predictive value of 28%.

Those who believe that treating the "index" cancer is sufficient, and are willing to ignore small nonindex cancers, have argued that these eligibility criteria were too stringent. Therefore, we have considered two other definitions of suitability when the extent of cancer on the contralateral side was consistent with modified characterizations of insignificant or indolent cancer [10,11]. Using these more liberal definitions of suitability, which

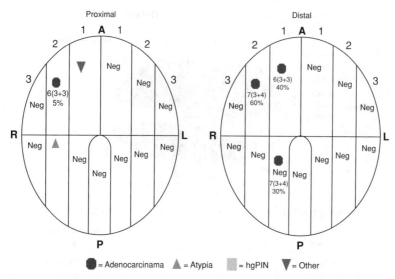

Figure 5.4 Sample prostate map. This illustrates the pathological findings after 3D-TPM.

allow potentially insignificant cancer on the side destined to be untreated, we still found that between 23% and 27% of patients presenting with unilateral small-volume cancer on office TRUS-biopsy were unsuitable for tissue-preserving therapy. In many patients by relying on repeat TRUS-biopsy alone, high-risk cancer on the side destined to be untreated would have been missed and in some this "untreated" side harbored the more aggressive cancer or so called "index" lesion. In the latter group, a focal therapy treatment plan that relied solely on repeat TRUS-biopsy could theoretically have targeted the "wrong" side. While our results imply a clear superiority of 3D-TPM over repeat TRUS-biopsy, a word of caution is needed, as there were several biases favoring 3D-TPM in this study, including the limited number of repeat TRUS-biopsy cores taken (average of 10/patient) in this study. Arguably, a saturation TRUS-biopsy scheme would have provided a fairer comparison as discussed above, and implied by ex vivo studies [12]. However, as recently demonstrated by Delongchamps et al. [13], merely increasing the number of TRUS-biopsy cores may not solve the inherent weakness of TRUS-biopsy; indeed, a 36-core biopsy scheme appeared to offer no advantage over an 18-core scheme. This is likely to be due to the inherent systematic error of undersampling anterior and apical areas of the prostate as well as clustering of sampling cores in the same peripheral zone areas when using the transrectal route.

On the basis of our own experience, validated by others, reliance on TRUS-biopsy to select patients for focal therapy may lead to an unacceptable failure rate, given the potential for significant cancer remaining

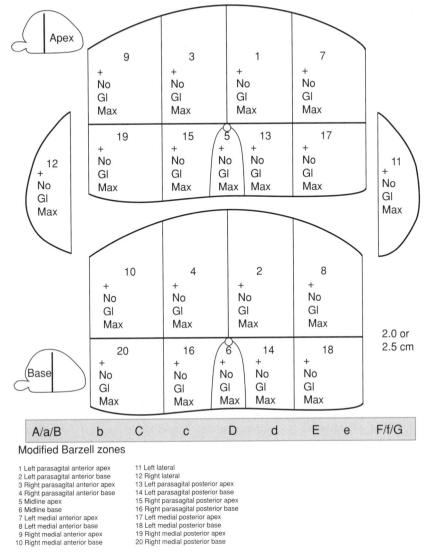

Modified Barzell zones

1 Left parasagital anterior apex	11 Left lateral
2 Left parasagital anterior base	12 Right lateral
3 Right parasagital anterior apex	13 Left parasagital posterior apex
4 Right parasagital anterior base	14 Left parasagital posterior base
5 Midline apex	15 Right parasagital posterior apex
6 Midline base	16 Right parasagital posterior base
7 Left medial anterior apex	17 Left medial posterior apex
8 Left medial anterior base	18 Left medial posterior base
9 Right medial anterior apex	19 Right medial posterior apex
10 Right medial anterior base	20 Right medial posterior base

Figure 5.5   UCL-modified Barzell zones. The University College London group use a 20 zone 3D-TPM system modified from the Barzell zones shown in Figure 5.3. (Courtesy of Hashim U. Ahmed, University College London.)

undetected and thereby untreated. When significant cancer is missed by TRUS-biopsy, in our experience the sites most commonly overlooked are the anterior apical regions of the prostate, a finding confirmed by Taira et al. [14]. Since the consequences of improper designation of a patient as a candidate for tissue preservation may be profound, we believe that 3D-TPM should be an integral component of any focal therapy program.

Conclusions

Until such time that newer imaging modalities can more accurately and reliably identify small foci of prostate cancer, 3D-TPM offers an accuracy in tumor localization that is not only crucial for proper patient selection and treatment planning (9–13), but also for follow-up biopsy validation of the efficacy of focal ablation, especially when considering novel technologies. Key to the success of tissue preserving treatments is proper patient selection. Currently, this is best achieved by a restaging procedure that can exclude patients with cancer outside the area destined to be treated while precisely locating the targeted area to be selectively ablated. A restaging procedure that uses 3D-TPM fulfills these criteria optimally fulfills these goals.

References

1. Eskew LA, et al. Systematic 5 region prostate biopsy is superior to sextant method for diagnosing carcinoma of the prostate. *J Urol* 1997;157(1): 199–202.
2. Jones JS. Saturation biopsy for detecting and characterizing prostate cancer. *BJU Int* 2007;99(6): 1340–1344.
3. Jones JS, et al. Saturation technique does not improve cancer detection as an initial prostate biopsy strategy. *J Urol* 2006;175(2): 485–488.
4. Megwalu, II, et al. Evaluation of a novel precision template-guided biopsy system for detecting prostate cancer. *BJUInt* 2008;102(5): 546–550.
5. Barzell WE, Melamed MR. Appropriate patient selection in the focal treatment of prostate cancer: The role of transperineal 3-dimensional pathologic mapping of the prostate—A 4-year experience. *Urology* 2007;70(6A): 27–35.
6. Barzell WE, Whitmore WF III. Transperineal template guided saturation biopsy of the prostate: rationale, indications, and technique. *Urol Times* 2003;31: 41–42.
7. Onik G, et al. Three-dimensional prostate mapping biopsy has a potentially significant impact on prostate cancer management. *JCO* 2009;27(26): 4321–4326.
8. Crawford ED, Barqawi A. Targeted focal therapy: a minimally invasive ablation technique for early prostate cancer. *Oncology (Williston Park)* 2007;21(1): 27–32.
9. Merrick GS, et al. The morbidity of transperineal template-guided prostate mapping biopsy. *BJUInt* 2008;101(12): 1524–1529.
10. Goto Y, et al. Distinguishing clinically important from unimportant prostate cancers before treatment: value of systematic biopsies. *J Urol* 1996;156(3): 1059–1063.
11. Epstein JI, et al. Pathologic and clinical findings to predict tumor extent of nonpalpable (stage T1c) prostate cancer. *JAMA* 1994;271(5): 368–374.
12. Epstein JI, et al. Utility of saturation biopsy to predict insignificant cancer at radical prostatectomy. *Urology* 2005;66(2): 356–360.
13. Delongchamps NB, et al. Saturation biopsies on autopsied prostates for detecting and characterizing prostate cancer. *BJUInt* 2009;103(1): 49–54.
14. Taira AV, et al. Performance of transperineal template-guided mapping biopsy in detecting prostate cancer in the initial and repeat biopsy setting. *Prostate Cancer Prostatic Dis* 2010;13(1): 71–77.

CHAPTER 6

Localization of Cancer within the Gland: Ultrasound Imaging

Ulrich Scheipers PhD

TomTec Imaging Systems GmbH, Unterschleissheim, Germany
Ruhr-University Bochum, Bochum, Germany

Introduction

Transrectal ultrasound imaging (TRUS) based on conventional B-mode (brightness mode) ultrasound is relatively insensitive because it rarely detects small well-differentiated tumors of sizes less than 0.1 cm^3. Using B-mode ultrasound, approximately two-thirds of all larger tumors can be seen, whereas the remainder appear isoechoic so cannot be identified as cancer.

Furthermore, B-mode ultrasound can be applied in different ways. The best diagnostic results are achieved when it is applied in a dynamic manner, which means that the gland is compressed manually during the examination by a light force by moving the transducer probe slightly toward and away from the gland. As the insonified prostate moves and changes its shape under varying compressions, equivalent to the concept of digital palpation, different tissue pathologies may be detected by the sharp eye. Thus, improved detection rates in comparison to the static application of B-mode ultrasound alone are possible.

Higher frequency probes that allow higher resolution images may lead to improved B-mode images in the future. Also, advanced imaging modalities such as harmonic imaging might help improve detection rates. It remains to be shown, if 3D-ultrasound modes can improve prostate cancer detection. The major advantage of B-mode ultrasound, especially when compared to the more complex modalities discussed below, is its general availability and relative inexpensiveness.

Focal Therapy in Prostate Cancer, First Edition. Edited by Hashim U Ahmed, Manit Arya, Peter Carroll and Mark Emberton.
© 2012 Blackwell Publishing Ltd. Published 2012 by Blackwell Publishing Ltd.

Elastography

An exciting and still relatively new diagnostic modality is ultrasound elastography or transrectal real-time elastography (TRTE), which is also known under the name of *strain* imaging (Figure 6.1). Elastography actually visualizes the local stiffness of the gland. While manual compression is applied to the insonified organ by slightly moving the ultrasound transducer toward and away from the gland, series of images are acquired at different compression ratios. The strain ratio or local stiffness is then visualized using specific color-coded images. The applied strain is typically in the range of a few percent of the insonified organ and too low to be uncomfortable to the patient. Besides the local elasticity value, i.e., the color, the regional homogeneity, or texture and prominent contours and seams within the image may pinpoint cancerous tissue.

First described by Ophir et al. [1], elastography was introduced to prostate detection by Lorenz et al. [2,3]. The first clinical results were based on a study of 404 patients [4] demonstrating a sensitivity of 84%. In a further study involving 492 men, elastography-guided biopsy was compared to systematic biopsy and showed a sensitivity of 86% and specificity of 72% [5]. Other studies with varying number of men have shown sensitivity ranging from 68% to 84% [6–9].

Elastography is used today as an adjunct to B-mode ultrasound in certain clinics. Although the results reported in several clinical studies are quite promising, elastography has not yet been widely introduced into clinical practice.

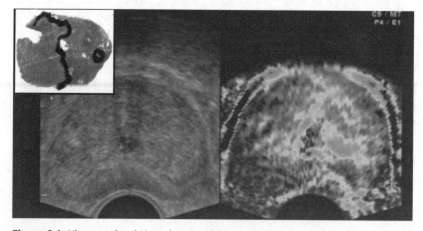

Figure 6.1 Ultrasound real-time elastography or strain imaging. Prostate cancer can hardly be detected using the conventional B-mode image alone. The strain image or elastogram on the right depicts stiff areas in red to black. Soft areas are colored yellow to blue. (See Plate 6.1.)

One feature that B-mode ultrasound and elastography have in common is the dependence of the results on the physician or sonographer conducting the examination. Experienced physicians and sonographers have higher prediction rates than novice physicians or sonographers due to learning curve issues. Ultrasound scanners supporting elastography are available from almost all major ultrasound companies, although most are restricted to linear probes, despite there being no known technical problems using the same software with transrectal probes.

Doppler and contrast-enhanced ultrasound

The use of contrast-enhanced ultrasound (CEUS) for prostate diagnostics has been investigated in clinical studies with only small patient numbers [10]. Sedelaar et al. discovered that the microvessel density (MVD) might be an indicative factor for prostate cancer, but the results of only seven patients were not representative enough to provide a final judgment on whether CEUS aids the detection of prostate cancer [11].

Borgers et al. evaluated contrast-enhanced 3D power Doppler ultrasound on 18 men with targeted biopsies to areas of suspicion [12]. A sensitivity of 85% for contrast-enhanced Doppler in comparison to 38% without was reported. Specificities were 85% for enhanced and 80% for baseline. In another study, Halpern et al. reported that detection of isoechoic tumors that were difficult to detect with conventional B-mode ultrasound benefited from contrast enhancement [13]. Subsequently, the same group evaluated CEUS on 60 men and reported a sensitivity of 65% compared with a sensitivity of 38% using B-mode and Doppler ultrasound [14]. Specificities were almost equivalent to 80% and 83%, respectively. Roy et al. evaluated 85 men using CEUS in combination with conventional B-mode and Doppler ultrasound [15]. Without CEUS, sensitivity of Doppler ultrasound alone was only 54%, but increased to 93% after contrast. Specificity increased from 79% to 87%. In a screening study involving 380 patients, Pelzer et al. compared systematic biopsy alone with a combination of systematic biopsy and contrast-enhanced color Doppler ultrasound for biopsy guidance [16]. The combination of both biopsy methods was 3.1 times more likely to detect prostate cancer than systematic biopsy alone. In a similar screening study Frauscher et al. evaluated 230 men [17] with systematic biopsy together with contrast-enhanced Doppler ultrasound-targeted biopsy; they showed that the latter modality was 2.6 times more likely to detect prostate cancer than systematic ultrasound-guided biopsy alone. In a study of 282 men using three-dimensional-reconstructed power Doppler ultrasound in comparison to conventional B-mode ultrasound sensitivity of power Doppler ultrasound was reported to be 92% and specificity 72%, in comparison to a sensitivity of 89% and specificity of 58% for B-mode ultrasound alone [18].

Ongoing opposition toward the wide use of contrast agents by the Food and Drug Agency in the United States is still delaying many efforts to further investigate this modality. Despite the promising results of the initial studies, the additional costs of the examination also have to be considered. In addition, giving contrast might prolong examination time, whereas Doppler ultrasound and elastography will only slightly prolong the time used for examination.

Sonohistology

Sonohistology, Histoscanning, or simply ultrasound tissue characterization is based on the extraction of local statistical parameters of tissue. Typically, complex mathematical models are applied to the raw ultrasound radio-frequency data, localizing areas within the gland that show a high statistical probability of being malignant. These areas are then depicted in graphical maps of the prostate or colored overlays fused with conventional B-mode ultrasound images (Figure 6.2).

On a technical level, systems for ultrasound tissue characterization usually comprise four main processing stages; ultrasound data acquisition, statistical parameter extraction, classification, and visualization [19]. Numerous ways of extracting tissue-describing parameters originating from different parameter groups have been described in the literature. Early approaches were based on video data acquisition. In the early stages of research, some groups characterized prostate tissue by evaluating single statistical parameters, e.g., ultrasound attenuation [20] or backscatter or by combining different parameters using a linear approach or a nearest

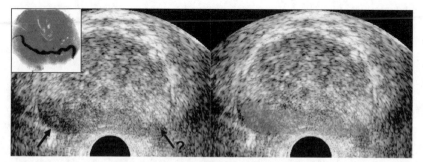

Figure 6.2 Ultrasound tissue characterization. Areas of the prostate exhibiting high cancer probability are marked in red. Not only the right part of the tumor (arrow) was highlighted by the classification system but nearly the whole extension of the cancerous region was also detected. (See Plate 6.2.)

neighbor technique [21]. Some groups also used nonlinear methods such as Kohonen maps [22] and conventional neural networks [23] to combine tissue parameters.

In an early study, Basset et al. analyzed video data originating from 16 men by means of texture parameters. However, the regions of interest applied in the study were too large to allow focal detection. An accuracy of 78% was reported [24]. Giesen et al. reported on analyzing video data acquired from 12 patients with images again analyzed using texture parameters. A sensitivity of 75% and specificity 78% were reported using needle biopsy results as the gold standard [25]. In a similar study, on the basis of the same system, Huynen et al. reported a sensitivity of 81% and specificity of 77%, which was achieved on a dataset originating from 51 patients [26]. Schmitz et al. analyzed radio-frequency data originating from 33 men using Kohonen maps as nonlinear classifiers showing a sensitivity of 82% and specificity of 88% [22]. Another group evaluated datasets originating from 21 patients using a nonlinear classifier based on fuzzy inference systems with four different statistical parameters. Overall classification rates estimated, as the area under the receiver operating characteristic (ROC) curve was 0.61 for isoechoic and 0.69 for hypoechoic and hyperechoic tumors. Histological whole-mount prostatectomy was used as the gold standard [27]. Loch et al. analyzed video data of 61 patients using various parameters and neural network classifiers eventually demonstrating a sensitivity of 79% and 99% specificity [28]. In several extensive publications, Feleppa et al. reported on the analysis of radio-frequency data. During the first few years of research, lookup tables were used to evaluate the data, but neural networks were used later [23]. Balaji et al. reported on a clinical study including data from 215 patients applying the tissue characterization software developed by Feleppa et al. An area under the ROC curve of 0.80 was reported when using needle biopsy results as the gold standard [29]. Scheipers et al. evaluated a network-based fuzzy inference system for classification. Several statistical parameters were combined to produce spatially resolved maps. In addition to two-dimensional maps, the output of the tissue characterization system was also rendered to yield volume reconstructions of the prostate and of carcinoma within the prostate. The ROC curve area was between 0.84 and 0.86 [30,31]. The latest and very promising results have been published by Braeckman et al. [32,33], who report a sensitivity of 95% for cancer lesions >0.2 cm^2 and a sensitivity of 100% for cancer lesions >0.5 cm^2, both at a specificity of 82%. A relatively small dataset originating from 29 patients has been evaluated for the study. However, the study is based on the only currently available commercial system for ultrasound tissue characterization of the prostate. After many years of research in this challenging field, further studies using larger patient numbers will hopefully follow.

Some early approaches used video data for tissue characterization. By using video data instead of radio-frequency or raw data, only a small set of tissue characterization parameters can be evaluated, which do not contain the necessary amount of information to classify the underlying tissue with sufficient accuracy. Only the use of radio-frequency or raw data can provide the information used to calculate parameters that characterize prostate tissue in a satisfactory way. Also, some of the works mentioned above use linear classifiers. As different parameters encountered in tissue characterization sometimes have a highly nonlinear interdependence, only a nonlinear model is considered to be able to combine these parameters and, thus, lead to reliable classification results. The major downside of ultrasound tissue characterization is its tremendous hunger for computational performance. The currently available approaches are far from real-time. Evaluation of a prostate dataset, which typically consists of a number of ultrasound images, still takes between several minutes and 1 hour. This means that the physician has to acquire ultrasound data, and then wait for the results of the system before starting the biopsy procedure. Future work will have to focus on increasing the performance of the systems alongside developments in image registration, in order to gain higher acceptance of tissue characterization.

Conclusion

The major challenge of conventional B-mode ultrasound for the detection of prostate cancer is the interobserver variability. A highly trained physician or sonographer may be able to detect the majority of tumors, especially when using ultrasound in a dynamic way, while a novice physician or sonographer may overlook small focal lesions or tumors with isoechoic properties.

Elastography enables the user to actually see differences in stiffness within the gland with his very own eyes. A specific color map or gray scale is used to visualize the local stiffness of the insonified tissue. Similar to the concept of digital palpation, stiff areas represent a high probability for cancer. Although elastography software is currently widely available, only a few systems allow elastography to be used in conjunction with transrectal probes.

Contrast-enhanced ultrasound for the detection and localization of prostate cancer is a very promising modality that still suffers from the ongoing discussions about the general safety of contrast agents. Encouraging results have been reported in several studies and further investigation is highly recommended. Ultrasound scanners that support specific contrast modes are widely available.

Ultrasound tissue characterization can to a certain degree automate the process of finding suspicious regions within the gland and hence reduce the gap in diagnostic results between expert and novice physicians and sonographers. Since ultrasound tissue characterization even evaluates characteristics of the ultrasound signal that cannot be seen in the conventional B-mode image, the approach may also be of great help to the expert. However, ultrasound tissue characterization software is not yet widely available and its use is therefore limited to research sites.

References

1. Ophir J, et al. A quantitative method for imaging the elasticity of biological tissues. Ultrason Imaging 1991;13: 111–134.
2. Lorenz A, et al. A new system for the acquisition of ultrasonic multicompression strain images of the human prostate in vivo. *Trans Ultras Ferro Freq Contr* 1999;46(5): 1147–1154.
3. Pesavento A, et al. A time-efficient and accurate strain estimation concept for ultrasonic elastography using iterative phase zero estimation. *Trans Ultras Ferro Freq Contr* 1999;46(5): 1057–1066.
4. König K, et al. Initial experiences with real-time elastography guided biopsies of the prostate. *J Urol* 2005;174: 115–117.
5. Pallwein L, et al. Sonoelastography of the prostate: comparison with systematic biopsy Findings in 492 patients. *Eur J Rad* 2008;65(2): 304–310.
6. Pallwein L, et al. Real-time elastography for detecting prostate cancer: Preliminary experience. *BJUInt* 2007;100(1): 42–46.
7. Tsutsumi M, et al. The impact of real-time tissue elasticity imaging (Elastography) on the detection of prostate cancer: Clinicopathological analysis. *Int J Clin Oncol* 2007;12: 250–255.
8. Salomon G, et al. Evaluation of prostate cancer detection with ultrasound real-time elastography: a comparison with step section pathological analysis after radical prostatectomy. *Eur Urol* 2008;54(6): 1209–1454.
9. Kamoi K, et al. The utility of transrectal real-time elastography in the diagnosis of rostate cancer. *Ultrasound Med Biol* 2008;34(7): 1025–1032.
10. Roy C, et al. Contrast enhances color Doppler endorectal sonography of prostate: Efficiency for detecting peripheral zone tumors and role for biopsy procedure. *J Urol* 2003;170(1): 69–72.
11. Sedelaar JPM, et al. Microvessel density: Correlation between contrast ultrasonography and histology of prostate cancer. *Eur Urol* 2001;40: 285–293.
12. Bogers HA, et al. Contrast-enhanced three-dimensional power Doppler angiography of the human prostate: Correlation with biopsy outcome. *Urology* 1999;54(1): 97–104.
13. Halpern EJ, et al. Initial experience with contrast-enhanced sonography of the prostate. *AJR* 2000;174: 1575–1580.
14. Halpern EJ, et al. Prostate cancer: Contrast-enhanced US for detection. *Radiology* 2001;219: 219–225.
15. Roy C, et al. Contrast enhances color Doppler endorectal sonography of prostate: Efficiency for detecting peripheral zone tumors and role for biopsy procedure. *J Urol* 2003;170(1): 69–72.

16. Pelzer A, et al. Prostate cancer detection in men with prostate specific antigen 4 to 10 ng/ml using a combined approach of contrast enhanced color Doppler targeted and systematic biopsy. *J Urol* 2005;173(6): 1926–1929.

17. Frauscher F, et al. Comparison of contrast enhanced color Doppler targeted biopsy with conventional systematic biopsy: Impact on prostate cancer detection. *J Urol* 2002;167(4): 1648–1652.

18. Sauvain JL, et al. Value of power Doppler and 3D vascular sonography as a method for diagnosis and staging of prostate cancer. *Eur Urol* 2003;44(1): 1–164.

19. Scheipers U. *Sonohistology—Methods and Systems for Ultrasonic Tissue Characterization based on a Multifeature Approach and Fuzzy Inference Systems.* Logos, Berlin; 2005.

20. Jenderka KV, et al. Tissue characterization by imaging the local frequency dependent relative backscatter coefficient, ultrasonic imaging and signal processing. Proceedings. SPIE 2000;3982: 270–277.

21. Feleppa EJ, et al. Ultrasonic spectral-parameter imaging of the prostate. *Int J Imag Sys Tech* 1997;8(1): 11–25.

22. Schmitz G, et al. Tissue characterization and imaging of the prostate using radio frequency ultrasonic signals. *Trans Ultras Ferro Freq Contr* 1999;46: 126–138.

23. Feleppa EJ, et al. Recent advances in ultrasonic tissue-type imaging of the prostate: improving detection and evaluation. *Acoustical Imaging 2007.* M.P. Andre ed. Springer, Dordrecht, 28: pp. 331–339.

24. Basset O, et al. Texture analysis of ultrasonic images of the prostate by means of cooccurrence matrices. *Ultrason Imaging* 1993;15: 218–237.

25. Giesen RJB, et al. Computer Analysis of transrectal ultrasound images of the prostate for the detection of carcinoma: A prospective study in radical prostatectomy Specimens. *J Urol* 1995;154: 1397–1400.

26. Huynen AL, et al. Analysis of ultrasonographic prostate images for the detection of prostatic carcinoma: The automated urologic diagnostic expert system. *Ultrasound Med Biol* 1994;20(1): 1–10.

27. Lorenz A, et al. Ultrasonic Tissue characterization—Assessment of prostate tissue malignancy in vivo using a conventional classifier based tissue classification approach and elastographic imaging. *Pro Ultrasonics Sym* 2000;2000: 1845–1848.

28. Loch T, et al. Artificial neural network analysis (ANNA) of prostatic transrectal ultrasound. *Prostate* 1999;39: 198–204.

29. Balaji KC, et al. Role of advanced 2 and 3-dimensional ultrasound for detecting prostate cancer. *J Urol* 2002;168: 2422–2425.

30. Scheipers U, et al. Ultrasonic tissue characterization for prostate diagnostics: Spectral parameters vs. texture parameters. *Biomed Tech* 2003;48(5): 122–129.

31. Scheipers U, et al. Ultrasonic multifeature tissue characterization for prostate diagnostics. *Ultrasound Med Biol* 2003;29(8): 1137–1149.

32. Braeckman J, et al. The accuracy of transrectal ultrasonography supplemented with computer-aided ultrasonography for detecting small prostate cancers. *BJUInt* 2008;102(11): 1560–1565.

33. Braeckman J, et al. Computer-aided ultrasonography (HistoScanning): A novel technology for locating and characterizing prostate cancer. *BJUInt* 2007;101(3): 293–298.

CHAPTER 7

Localization of Cancer within the Prostate: Dynamic Contrast-Enhanced MRI

Philippe Puech MD PhD[1,2], Anwar Padhani FRCR[3], Laurent Lemaitre MD PhD[4], Nacim Betrouni PhD[2], Pierre Colin MD[5], and Arnauld Villers MD PhD[5]

[1] CHRU Lille, University of Lille Nord de France, Lille, France
[2] INSERM, University of Lille Nord de France, Lille, France
[3] Mount Vernon Cancer Centre, Northwood, Middlesex, UK
[4] Department of Radiology, University of Lille Nord de France, Lille, France
[5] Department of Urology, CHRU Lille, University of Lille Nord de France, Lille, France

Introduction

Multiparametric MRI has emerged as the method of choice for prostate cancer localization. Numerous studies have shown that morphological T2-weighted (T2W) imaging needs to be combined with one or more functional techniques such as diffusion-weighted imaging (DW-MRI), dynamic contrast-enhanced MRI (DCE-MRI), and magnetic resonance proton spectroscopic imaging (MRSI) for this purpose. The rationale for the combination approach is that each technique highlights different biological or physical characteristics of prostatic tissue which, when considered alone is insufficient for accurate localization of prostate cancer.

Mirowitz et al. first demonstrated contrast medium enhancement for delineating prostate anatomy and detecting seminal vesicle invasion, and reported increased enhancement of prostatic carcinoma [1]. Soon there after, Brown et al. showed that the intraprostatic extent of cancer was better demonstrated when contrast medium was injected at the same time as the patient was being scanned [2]. They ascribed their findings to known increased vascularity of tumors. Thereafter, the first dynamic MRI experiments were described wherein serial T1-weighted (T1W) imaging sequences were acquired before, during, and after contrast injection; these works depicted prostate cancer hypervascularization during the first

Focal Therapy in Prostate Cancer, First Edition. Edited by Hashim U Ahmed, Manit Arya, Peter Carroll and Mark Emberton.
© 2012 Blackwell Publishing Ltd. Published 2012 by Blackwell Publishing Ltd.

pass of contrast [3]. Subsequently, the use of DCE-MRI technique for improving prostate cancer imaging has been widely described, not only for (a) local staging and (b) identifying suspicious areas in the gland before treatment but also for (c) detecting recurrences after external beam radiotherapy (EBRT) or radical prostatectomy (RP) [4].

Importantly, a variety of methods have been used for analyzing DCE images, ranging from simple visual reading of images and enhancement curve shapes [5], to complex computer-assisted analyses of time–signal-intensity curves with pharmacokinetic modeling [6], many requiring analyses of arterial input function (AIF) for their implementation. Although optimal clinical usage has yet to be defined, DCE-MRI has made the transition from research to clinical practice, and is now an easily accessible technique that can be performed in just a few minutes, using any MRI device.

Pathophysiological basis

Several studies have demonstrated that malignant tumors have focal areas of higher microvessel densities than corresponding normal tissues. Anarchic, poorly differentiated, and fragile capillaries are found within tumors, with leaky interendothelial junctions that favor extravasation of plasma into the extravascular, extracellular space (EES). Thus, tumor vessels are hyperperfused and hyperpermeable compared with normal tissues and it is this property that DCE-MRI exploits for generating image contrast.

DCE-MRI sequences require a bolus intravenous injection of a low-molecular-weight paramagnetic contrast agent (usually 0.1mmol/kg body weight (BW)). During the first pass of the contrast bolus in the capillary bed, the concentration of gadolinium chelate reaches a peak. Contrast agent rapidly crosses the vascular endothelium to enter the EES, where the concentration is zero (Figure 7.1). Enhancement becomes detectable on T1W images as the contrast agent interacts with water molecules in the EES changing their relaxation rates. Since the contrast agent does not enter the intracellular space, interactions with intracellular water are more limited but do nevertheless occur as water diffuses into and out of cells. Contrast agent remains in the EES as long as the concentration there is below or equal to that in the vascular space. As blood contrast agent concentration falls (due to excretion and whole-body redistribution) so the EES concentration falls with gadolinium molecules migrating from the EES to the vascular space. This is called the "wash-out" phase.

Thus, the time–signal-intensity curve observed during a DCE-MRI sequence exhibits a baseline signal initially, then a fast "wash-in" corresponding to the arrival of contrast medium and leakage into EES (Figure 7.1). This wash-in phase is followed by a plateau phase, when the

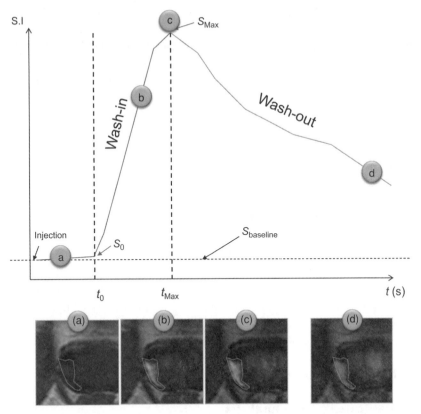

Figure 7.1 Illustration of a typical peripheral zone cancer during the different steps of its enhancement in a DCE-MRI sequence (approximately 5 minutes). The time–signal-intensity curve is computed for the mean voxel intensity within the dotted region of interest. Baseline signal intensity (a) of the unenhanced prostate is observed from the time when the contrast medium is injected into the brachial vein to its arrival in the capillaries of the region of interest at t_0. Thereafter, the contrast medium rapidly enters the extravascular extracellular space (EES) during the "wash-in" phase (b), reaching a peak concentration (c). This is followed by a signal decrease corresponding to the migration of the contrast medium from the EES to the vascular space. This process takes place more or less slowly, depending mainly on endothelial membrane permeability, blood flow, and the amount of contrast agent that has accumulated. This is called the "wash-out" phase (d). When the pace of migration is particularly slow, acquisition can be too short to demonstrate it, and the wash-out phase takes on a plateau-like appearance.

EES and vascular spaces have equivalent concentrations, then a wash-out phase. The speed of enhancement, peak level reached, and rate of wash-out are dependent on multiple factors, including tissue factors (perfusion, permeability, EES volume), patient factors (hydration, hematocrit), characteristics of the contrast agent (concentration, relaxivity, volume, injection speed), and also machine setup factors (sequence parameters, gain, scaling factors). Regardless, DCE-MRI does reveal the most vascularized areas of the prostate gland with prostate cancer appearing as an area of higher wash-in and wash-out rates than normal tissue. Occasionally, benign pathologies such as hyperplastic stromal nodules in the transition zone, inflammation, and even normal tissue after biopsy can sometimes have high wash-in and wash-out rates. Thus, there is considerable overlap of contrast enhancement patterns between benign and malignant tissue, which emphasizes the need to interpret DCE-MRI characteristics with corresponding morphological patterns depicted on the DCE-MRI and by other techniques, including T2W and DWI-MRI imaging.

Enhancement analysis

In routine practice, protocols must include the whole gland. Imaging is performed using variants of gradient echo T1W sequences, in either two-dimensional or three-dimensional. Images are usually acquired at a lower resolution than T2W images, but in the same plane to facilitate image synchronization and multiparametric analysis. There are three different classes of technique described for analyzing contrast medium uptake in the gland, depending on the purpose of the MRI examination (cancer detection, staging, treatment planning, or follow-up).

Visual (qualitative) analysis

The simplest way of reviewing a DCE-MRI dataset is as a movie using either the raw images or serial subtraction images, noting the onset of enhancement, its focality, symmetry, and thereafter the progressive increase of enhancement as more and more contrast agent arrives at the tissue level. It is the speed of onset of enhancement that is usually the most informative to detect suspicious areas. Image contrast can be emphasized by image subtraction, when motion artifacts are limited. Fat suppression can be useful for detecting seminal vesicle and tumor spread beyond the capsule. It can also be useful for monitoring the effects of focal therapy in the periprostatic fat or in surrounding structures (muscles, rectum, sphincter). This basic review method is available in all centers, and no additional software or posttreatment application is necessary. However, while it can be used to detect lesions with significant wash-in, it cannot be used to adequately analyze the wash-out.

Curves (semiquantitative) analysis

Wash-out analysis requires some postprocessing software that enables regions of interest (ROIs) placement on visually detected suspicious areas and the display of time–signal-intensity curves. Depending on the curve shapes displayed interpretations can be made to help radiologists to distinguish malignant from benign tissues. The success of this ROI method is enhanced when combined with morphological features discussed in Section "Visual (qualitative) analysis" and both are recommended for the initial analysis of DCE-MRI.

Postprocessing software can also extract parameters from each curve in each voxel at a particular slice position. Parametric maps of onset time, time to peak, relative enhancement, and wash-in and wash-out rates can be generated; these may be useful for localizing the most suspicious areas of the gland. Computer-aided diagnosis (CAD) software can perform automatic analysis of the curves [7], in order to help distinguish malignant hypervascularized areas from benign ones. Semiquantitative parameters are relatively simple to implement, but have marked limitations, including the fact that the displayed results are highly dependent on experimental conditions, including injection flow rate, sequence parameters, and gain factors. Thus, semiquantitative parameters cannot be compared between centers and lack biological meaning in terms of explaining the underlying pathophysiology. Nevertheless, they are useful with some groups demonstrating that the best discriminators of prostate cancer were relative peak enhancement in the PZ and wash-out in the TZ [8,9].

Quantitative analysis

New techniques have been developed for extracting more comparable and reproducible pathophysiologically relevant parameters from the enhancement curves, many of which also take into account individual patient AIFs. All these techniques apply multicompartment pharmacokinetic models to the enhancement patterns observed. Numerous models have been described. The most widely used model is two-compartmental [10]. The two-compartmental model provides estimations of the volume transfer constant (K_{trans}; wash-in rate; unit min^{-1}), rate constant (k_{ep}; wash-out rate; unit min^{-1}), and the volume of EES per unit of tissue (ve; unit %). Recently, the two-compartmental model has been extended, yielding an additional plasma volume parameter (vp; unit %). These more physiologically relevant kinetic parameters have also been shown to help localize cancer within the prostate gland; but not unexpectedly, there is overlap between malignant tissues, benign pathologies, and normal tissues. The latter should not come as a surprise: the contrast agent used in DCE-MRI is of low molecular weight and readily crosses prostatic capillary membranes. Although quantitative analysis is time-consuming, requires expensive postprocessing software, and suffers from a cascade of assumptions (conversion of time–signal-intensity curves to medium concentration–time curves, arbitrary choice of the model used), it is only by the use of such techniques that reproducible intra- and interpatient parameters can be derived that are mandatory for assessing effects of therapies that target prostatic microvasculature.

Acquisition techniques

Prebiopsy MRI

Where possible, it is important to perform multiparametric MRI before undertaking prostatic biopsies. Postbiopsy hemorrhagic and inflammatory artifacts hinder DCE-MRI interpretation because the former appear as high-intensity areas that prevent enhancement detection. The biopsy procedure even in the absence of hemorrhage can induce reactive hyperemia, thus yielding abnormal enhancement even in normal tissues. Postbiopsy hemorrhage also has a significant impact on T2W, DW-MRI, and MRSI sequences, and can persist for 2–6 months. Consequently, these artifacts have a negative impact on the quality of the examinations and on lesion detection accuracy. The assessment of tumor burden and contours is important for deciding therapy, and postbiopsy hemorrhagic and inflammatory artefacts are impediments in this regard. Additionally, these artifacts hamper comparisons of repeated MRI examinations performed in the follow-up of conservative management. Thus, multiparametric MRI, especially if it includes DCE-MRI sequences, should ideally be performed either before or sometime after a biopsy [11,12].

MRI protocol

Acquisition can be carried out either using an external high-resolution pelvic phased-array (HR-PPA) coil or by using combined endorectal and high-resolution pelvic phased-array coils (ER-PPA). The use of the ERC alone is not recommended for DCE-MRI because the signal intensity may be too low in the anterior part of the gland, and because cancer detection is best when the signal intensity is homogeneous across the imaging field of view.

Dynamic contrast-enhanced imaging is performed using spoiled gradient recalled echo (GRE) T1W sequences that can be either in two-dimensional or three-dimensional. There are numerous variants in acquisition parameters designed to increase the signal-to-noise ratio and temporal resolution (including parallel imaging, fat saturation, keyhole imaging) that are not always compatible with pharmacokinetic modeling. Generally, acquisition is performed in the same axial plane as T2W and DW-MRI. When further comparisons are needed, a reference acquisition plane is chosen, such as the axial oblique plane perpendicular to the rectal wall.

A typical quantitative 1.5T analysis protocol using a simple three-dimensional GRE sequence allows for the repetitive acquisition of 30 series of fifteen 4-mm slices every 10 seconds, with a total acquisition time of 5 minutes, using a 160-mm field of view, and a resolution of 0.8 × 0.7 × 4 mm. At 3T, the higher signal-to-noise ratio allows for shorter acquisition times, (e.g., only 7 seconds for a single volume of 15 slices) and thinner slices. Both protocols are compatible with quantitative analysis, as the latter requires high temporal resolution (2–10 seconds) rather than spatial resolution, due to the fact that calculated pharmacokinetic parameters may not be reliable beyond a resolution of 15 seconds. Contrast agent injection must be performed using an automatic injector, at a dose of 0.1mmol/kg BW and a rate of 2–3 mL/s, and flushed by normal saline given at the same rate, in order to produce reproducible bolus injections. An antiperistaltic may be given before the start of examination to suppress bowel movements.

Cancer detection

Importance of tumor mapping at diagnosis

Precise tumor mapping, including the location and extent of each suspicious area, is mandatory for guiding biopsies and, when cancer is confirmed, for selecting the best therapeutic option (active surveillance, radical or focalized treatment). For example, in the case of surgical treatment information from tumor mapping helps to avoid positive surgical margins and preserve the neurovascular bundles, bladder neck, and urethral sphincter. Tumor mapping is also extremely important when planning focal therapy (Figure 7.2).

Accuracy

Surprisingly, there have been very few studies documenting the ability of DCE-MRI to detect cancer foci in patients with elevated PSA and no proven cancer: in a series of 93 patients who underwent a repeat biopsy, Cheikh et al. [13] compared T2W and DCE images, both interpreted using visual criteria only. They found sensitivity values of 47.8% and 82.6%, respectively, with a specificity of 44.3% and 20%, in the per patient analysis, and a sensitivity of 32.1% and 52.4%, with a specificity of 89.7 and 83.5%, in the per sector analysis ($n = 10$). In most other studies, the ability of MRI to characterize a suspicious ROI is usually assessed in relation to RP [14–16]. This method of validation suffers from selection bias and many studies ignore smaller cancers (<0.5 cc).

Overall, DCE-MRI (including T2W imaging) has a sensitivity of 73–87%, a specificity of 79–93%, a negative predictive value of approximately 75%, and an area under the ROC curve (Az) of approximately 0.90. DCE-MRI increases the sensitivity of T2W imaging with a slight loss of specificity, thus resulting in greater accuracy (or Az) [17].

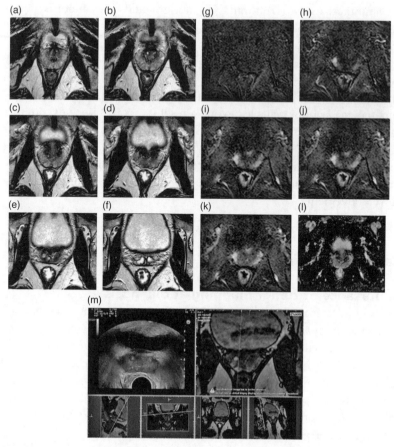

Figure 7.2 Patient with a history of slowly increasing PSA levels (currently 6.5 ng/mL) and two negative 12-core biopsies performed five (PSA 3.7 ng/mL in 2005) and 4 years earlier (PSA 4.4 ng/mL in 2006). DRE results were normal. A T2W MRI scan (images (a–f)) showed a small, 30-cc prostate, with diffuse homogeneous low signal intensity, but no suspicious lesion. A subtracted DCE-MRI scan performed on a 1.5T device equipped with an HRPPA coil revealed a significant 13 × 10 mm suspicious area in the right lateral base (images (g–k)) were taken in the same plane as image (d); (g) is unenhanced, (h) is the earliest enhanced image, and images (i–k) are subsequent enhanced images acquired every 15 seconds). A diffusion-weighted scan in the same plane as the lesion (image (l)) did not reveal any anomaly. All systematic posterior biopsies (12 cores) were negative, but both additional DCE-MRI-guided targeted biopsies under image fusion (m) were positive for adenocarcinoma (Gleason 3 + 4 = 7). (See Plate 7.2.)

DCE-MRI accuracy and cancer size

Several studies have also assessed the threshold volume of DCE-MRI for cancer detection. Using ERC and T2W imaging only, in a series of 70 patients, Roethke et al. concluded that MRI cannot exclude cancers below 0.4 cc, and has a high sensitivity above 20 mm (1.6 cc) [18]. Histological

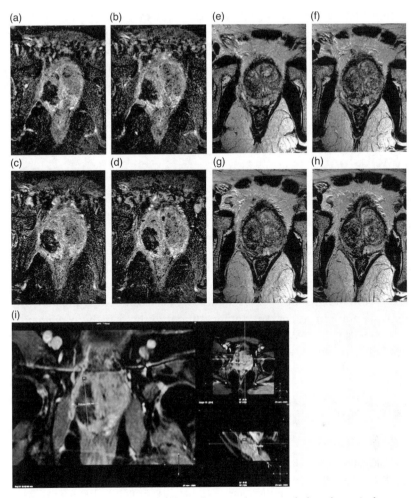

Figure 7.3 DCE-MRI performed 7 days after vascular-targeted photodynamic therapy
(VTP). The patient had an initial PSA of 8.3 ng/mL, with only one positive core out of
12 (Gleason 3 + 3 = 6) at biopsy, in the right median lobe. Images (a–d) show four
consecutive slices of the treated gland in a late (4 minutes postinjection)
three-dimensional DCE-MRI scan performed on a 1.5T device using an HRPPA coil and
fat saturation. They clearly show a well-circumscribed hypovascularized area
corresponding to the treated zone (right posterior lobe). Images (e–h) are
corresponding T2W slices, showing only large areas of low intensity, with unclear
margins. Image (i) illustrates the advantage of using multiplanar reconstruction to
assess treated areas. (See Plate 7.3.)

correlations have revealed a high sensitivity and specificity of DCE-MRI for
cancers with a volume greater than 0.5 cc (70). In a series of 83 patients
who underwent RP, Puech et al. showed that the mean volume of cancers
detected at DCE-MRI was 2.44 cc, with an Az of 0.87, 0.78, and 0.70 for
cancer foci >0.5 cc, >0.3 cc, and >0.2 cc, respectively [14].

Evaluation of focal treatment efficiency

Tissue necrosis efficiency can best be assessed using DCE-MRI, as areas of relative poor enhancement. In this way, it is possible to determine whether all or part of the target lesion has been treated and assess potential complications (extraprostatic, urethral, or rectal necrosis) (Figure 7.3) (see Chapter 16).

Conclusion

DCE-MRI has become a mainstream clinical tool with recognized indications in the imaging of prostate cancer. Current roles include lesion localization, staging (depiction of capsular penetration and seminal vesicle invasion) and the detection of suspected tumor recurrence following definitive treatment. Limitations of the technique include inadequate lesion characterization, particularly in differentiating prostatitis from cancer in the peripheral gland and distinguishing between benign prostatic hyperplasia and transition zone tumors. Importantly, it is the combination of DCE-MRI with T2W, DW-MRI and MRSI that yields the best diagnostic performance.

References

1. Mirowitz SA, et al. Evaluation of the prostate and prostatic carcinoma with gadolinium-enhanced endorectal coil MR imaging. *Radiology* 1993;186(1): 153–157.
2. Brown G, et al. The role of intravenous contrast enhancement in magnetic resonance imaging of prostatic carcinoma. *Clin Radiol* 1995;50(9): 601–606.
3. Jager GJ, et al. Dynamic TurboFLASH subtraction technique for contrast-enhanced MR imaging of the prostate: correlation with histopathologic results. *Radiology* 1997;203(3): 645–652.
4. Alonzi R, et al. Dynamic contrast enhanced MRI in prostate cancer. *EurJ of Radiol* 2007;63(3): 335–350.
5. Padhani AR, et al. Dynamic contrast enhanced MRI of prostate cancer: correlation with morphology and tumour stage, histological grade and PSA. *Clin Radiol* 2000;55(2): 99–109.
6. Tofts PS, et al. Estimating kinetic parameters from dynamic contrast-enhanced T(1)-weighted MRI of a diffusable tracer: standardized quantities and symbols. *J Magn Reson Imaging* 1999;10(3): 223–232.
7. Puech P, et al. Computer-assisted diagnosis of prostate cancer using DCE-MRI data: design, implementation and preliminary results. *Int J Comput Assist Radiol Surg* 2009;4(1): 1–10.
8. Engelbrecht MR, et al. Discrimination of prostate cancer from normal peripheral zone and central gland tissue by using dynamic contrast-enhanced MR imaging. *Radiology* 2003;229(1): 248–254.

9. Futterer JJ, et al. Prostate cancer localization with dynamic contrast-enhanced MR imaging and proton MR spectroscopic imaging. *Radiology* 2006;241(2): 449–458.

10. Ocak I, et al. Dynamic contrast-enhanced MRI of prostate cancer at 3 T: a study of pharmacokinetic parameters. *AJR* 2007;189(4): 849.

11. Ahmed HU, et al. Is it time to consider a role for MRI before prostate biopsy? *Nat Rev Clin Oncol* 2009;6(4): 197–206.

12. Villers A, et a. Dynamic contrast enhanced, pelvic phased arraly magnetic resonance imaging of localized prostate cancer for predicting tumor volume: correlation with radical prostatectomy findings. *J Urol* 2006;176(6 Pt 1): 2432–2437.

13. Cheikh AB, et al. Evaluation of T2-weighted and dynamic contrast-enhanced MRI in localizing prostate cancer before repeat biopsy. *Eur Radiol* 2009;19(3): 770–778.

14. Puech P, et al. Dynamic contrast-enhanced-magnetic resonance imaging evaluation of intraprostatic prostate cancer: correlation with radical prostatectomy specimens. *Urology* 2009;74(5): 1094–1099.

15. Nakashima J, et al. Endorectal MRI for prediction of tumor site, tumor size, and local extension of prostate cancer. *Urology* 2004;64(1): 101–105

16. Preziosi P, et al. Enhancement patterns of prostate cancer in dynamic MRI. *Eur Radiol* 2003;13(5): 925–930.

17. Kirkham AP, et al. How Good is MRI at detecting and characterising cancer within the prostate? *Euro Urol* 2006;50(6): 1163–1175.

18. Roethke MC, et al. Tumorsize dependent detection rate of endorectal MRI of prostate cancer-A histopathologic correlation with whole-mount sections in 70 patients with prostate cancer. *Eur J Radiol* 2010 Mar 11. [Epub ahead of print]

CHAPTER 8

Localization of Cancer within the Gland: Diffusion-Weighted Magnetic Resonance Imaging of the Prostate

Sophie F. Riches MPhys MSc, Nina Tunariu MD, and Nandita M. deSouza BSc MBBS MD FRCP FRCR

Institute of Cancer Research and Royal Marsden Hospital, London, UK

Introduction

Magnetic resonance imaging (MRI) using T2W contrast and an endorectal coil is currently the standard method of imaging prostate cancer. However, the sensitivity and specificity of T2W-MRI for localization within the gland varies from 60–82% to and 55–70%, respectively [1]. An alternative is to develop image contrast through "apparent diffusivity" because normal and tumor-containing tissue exhibits differences in microvascular and cellular content that result in differences in water movement within these tissues. DW-MRI exploits these differences to differentiate normal and cancer containing tissues (Figures 8.1 and 8.2). The values of the apparent diffusion coefficient (ADC), the quantitative parameter obtained from DW-MRI, have been correlated successfully with cell density in prostatectomy specimens [2]. In tumours, the use of DW-MRI immediately after treatment has been shown to be an early indicator of subsequent response as the measured ADC reflects the initial degree of cell swelling and extracellular edema.

Methodology

Imaging sequences
Single-shot echo planar imaging (EPI), which allows a whole slice to be imaged in a time-frame of a few seconds without artifact from respiratory

---

Focal Therapy in Prostate Cancer, First Edition. Edited by Hashim U Ahmed, Manit Arya, Peter Carroll and Mark Emberton.

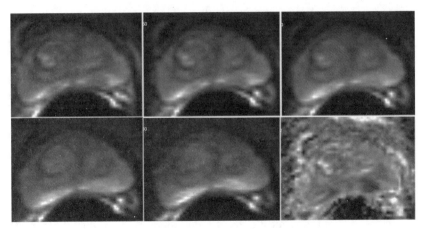

Figure 8.1 Diffusion-weighted endorectal prostate images in a 59-year-old man at *b*-values of (top row from left to right) 0, 100, 300 (bottom row from left to right), 500, and 800 s/mm, with corresponding ADC map (each optimally windowed). Dark regions of restricted diffusion on the ADC map are more easily seen than the corresponding persistently bright areas on the DW-MRI images.

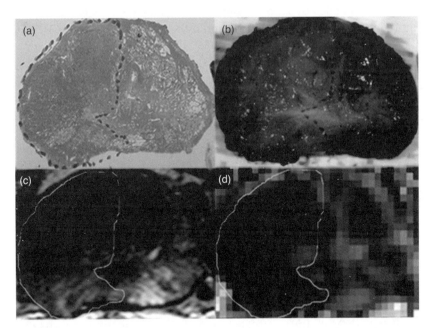

Figure 8.2 (a) Hematoxylin and eosin-stained histology section from a whole-mount prostatectomy specimen (b) showing tumor outline (in blue). On the T2W image in (c), this tumor outline (in yellow) has been warped to fit the T2W image slice and then overlaid onto the ADC map in (d). The tumor has lower ADC compared to the normal left peripheral zone. (See Plate 8.2.) (Reprinted with permission from Extra-Cranial Applications of Diffusion-Weighted MRI, Edited by Bachir Taouli, 2010, © Cambridge University Press)

motion, is the most commonly used prostate sequence. However, distortion due to local field heterogeneity, local fat causing chemical shift artifacts, and susceptibility artifacts from both the bone-tissue interfaces and air in balloon of the endorectal coils can be significant. This has prompted exploration of mean single shot fast spin echo (FSE) sequences, but these have reduced signal-to-noise ratio (SNR) and exhibit general blurring compared with EPI sequences.

The low bandwidth in the phase encoding direction of an EPI sequence can be problematic as periprostatic fat is within the field of view and causes a fat/water shift of ~8 pixels at 1.5-Tesla (1.5-T). Multishot EPI divides the acquisition into multiple segments that reduces the chemical shift and susceptibility artifacts by increasing the bandwidth at the expense of increased scan time. Eddy-currents generated by the diffusion gradient will result in spatial encoding errors, causing geometric distortions in the phase-encode directions. Phase-encoding wrap in small field-of-view images can be stopped using saturation bands applied on either side of the field of view allowing the echo time (TE) to be kept short. Due to the effectively infinite TR of an EPI sequence, the diffusion signal attenuation is compounded by T2-relaxation, and T2-shine through is evident on diffusion-weighted images, which should therefore be acquired with the shortest possible TE.

Images are acquired with multiple b-values (a parameter combining gradient strength and duration) and ADCs derived from the slope of signal intensity plotted against the b-values quantify the degree of restriction of water diffusion. Accurate derivation of the ADC is best performed by curve-fitting of the signal decay with several b-values, but the need to reduce the time cost of diffusion-imaging means two b-values are often employed to estimate the ADC, acquiring data with no diffusion gradient and at a single b-value. Errors associated with this estimation can be minimized by (a) increasing the SNR and (b) using a b-value in the diffusion-weighted image whose value is the reciprocal of the expected diffusion coefficient usually between ~550 and 1000 s/mm^2.

Studies have shown that ADC values decrease by >20% for normal tissue and >40% for malignant tissues when b-values of 2000 s/mm^2 are used, increasing the overlap in the ADC values of normal and malignant tissues [3]. However, for a constant number of signal averages, the ~20% reduction of SNR in prostate tissues at the higher b-values means that errors in the ADC are likely due to insufficient SNR for accurate data fitting, which can lead to underestimation of the ADC. In order to overcome this, some clinical scanners allow increased signal averages at higher b-value images, although the variable SNR associated with different b-values in the resulting signal decay curve must still be accounted for in parameter calculations.

Hardware

A rigid or balloon endorectal coil in close proximity to the prostate offers improved SNR over external coils [4], with more accurate ADC calculations from fast EPI sequences. The increased distortion visible with air-filled balloon coils (because of the air/tissue boundary) can be reduced by filling the coil with substances of similar susceptibility to tissue such as perfluorocarbon. Movement of the coil during high vibrations experienced with EPI sequences has been found to be limited locally by weighting the handle of the coil with a sandbag. The prostate exhibits periodic motion associated with peristalsis and respiration; peristalsis can be reduced with an intramuscular administration of hyoscine butylbromide. Respiratory motion occurs in the anterior-posterior direction so the phase-encoding direction should be chosen to avoid this axis.

As diffusion-weighted imaging is an inherently low SNR technique, the increased signal at 3.0-Tesla (3-T) magnetic field strength allows an increase in spatial resolution or a decrease in scan time (Figures 8.3 and 8.4). Pelvic array DW-MRI at 3 T can use parallel imaging techniques to reduce scan times and hence the resulting motion artifacts while maintaining the SNR level obtainable at 1.5 T; however, with low SNR inter- and intrasession reproducibility can be poor. Magnetic susceptibility artifacts and distortion are reported in the diffusion images from patients with dilated rectums when using pelvic array coils alone at 3 T, which are compounded by air-filled coils.

Analysis

The accuracy of two-point sampling schemes for derivation of ADC depends on the assumption that the signal decays monoexponentially with increasing b-values. However, it is proposed that at very low b-values the motion detected is dominated by the fast bulk motion associated with

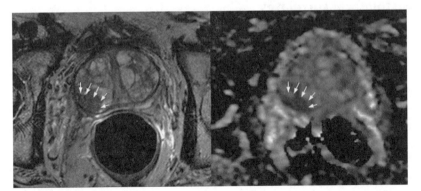

Figure 8.3   3-T T2W (left) and ADC map (right) of a 65-year-old man with tumor in the right midgland of the prostate. The increased SNR at 3 T allows more structure of the prostate to be seen in the ADC map, possibly allowing better tumor detection.

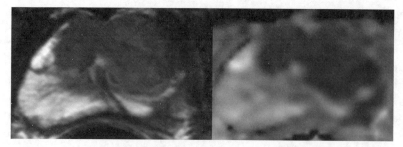

Figure 8.4   3-T T2W (left) and ADC map (right) of a 79-year-old man with tumor in the central gland of the prostate.

perfusion in the tissues. In order to remove the effect of the perfusion from the diffusion measurements, often three or more b-values are employed and the signal from the $b = 0$ s/mm^2 image is not used in the two-point calculation of the monoexponential ADC [5]. Data acquired using eleven b-values ranging from 0 s/mm^2 to 800 s/mm^2 showed that removing b-values less than 100 s/mm^2 from a monoexponential model resulted in the same ADC as predicted by a biexponential model that accounted for both the perfusion and diffusion components. Studies looking at biexponential modeling of prostate diffusion over an extended b-value range upto 3000 s/mm^2 postulate there are two distinct diffusion coefficients, one fast and one slow, but their possible origin is not understood. At these very high b-values, care must be taken to ensure that insufficient SNR does not cause monoexponential signal decay to appear biexponential because of the presence of irregularly distributed noise in magnitude data.

Utility of prostate DW—MRI in the clinic

Histological correlates

Defining tumor using T2W signal intensity and validating results against sextant biopsy or step-section histology have reported ADC values of prostate cancer to be significantly lower than in nonmalignant peripheral zone (PZ) [6–9]. Differences between tumor and normal central gland tissue have been more variable [10, 11]. ADC values obtained at 3 T for prostate cancer and normal PZ are similar to those acquired at 1.5 T. Most studies use T2W contrast or diffusion-weighted information to define the region of abnormality, thus biasing ADC values of tumors away from normal tissue values. The gold standard for determination of ADC values of tumor use histologically defined tumor and normal regions transposed onto the ADC maps by registering them with step-section histology. This methodology reveals a smaller difference between tumor and nontumor ADC values compared with previous studies. Differences between tumor and nontumor ADCs are more marked if tumors of less than 1 cm^2 cross section were excluded suggesting either partial volume effects or an inherent difference in diffusion in smaller tumors.

Value in tumor detection

On conventional T2W imaging, prostate cancer is mainly recognized as a focal low signal-intensity lesion within the PZ. However, such change also may arise as a result of an inflammatory process within the gland. Furthermore, malignant lesions isointense with peripheral zone may not be distinguished as tumor. DWI-MRI improves identification of tumor in these cases because of differences between tissue types [12]. The glandular normal prostate compared with the highly cellular regions encountered in prostate cancers where diffusion is restricted within reduced intracellular and interstitial spaces, produces a substantial differential in ADC. We reported that an experienced reader, using an endorectal 1.5-T MRI protocol, could improve the detection rate of tumor in patients on active surveillance from 46.5% to 71% by adding ADC maps in the evaluation [13]. Other authors also using an endorectal coil at 1.5 T have reported a sensitivity between 81% and 88% and specificity between 84% and 89% by using a combined T2W + ADC evaluation [14, 15]. Similar increases in tumor detection have been reported using pelvic phased-array coils at 1.5 T and 3 T.

ADC values derived from DWI can be used to separate nodules on the basis of their cellularity. The ADC values of malignant prostate nodules appear significantly lower than in nonmalignant prostate nodules. This has particular implications for identifying the 30% of cancers that arise within the central gland. Malignant nodules are typically more cellular than the nodules of BPH; there is significant heterogeneity in the latter where glandular, mixed, and stromal BPH nodules with different cellularity all coexist. It is this heterogeneity of DW-MRI within well-defined nodules in the central gland that identifies them as benign. Malignant central gland nodules are often more irregular, ill-defined, and homogeneously low in signal-intensity with mass effect.

Several authors have investigated the use of threshold ADC values in identifying tumor foci in the PZ. We found that using an ADC cutoff value of 0.0016 mm^2/s to differentiate malignant from nonmalignant PZ tissue gave a sensitivity of 86.7% and specificity of 72.7% [16]. Using a similar cutoff value, other authors have reported a sensitivity of 95% and specificity of 65% [17].

Detection of tumor recurrence after focal therapy

After focal-targeted therapy such as high-intensity focused ultrasound ablation (HIFU), cryoablation, and radiotherapy, there is a need for imaging techniques to establish completeness of the ablative therapy, get an early indication of longer term outcome and an early detection of tumor recurrence. The conclusion of small published single center studies coincide with our local expertise that the combination of anatomical (preferably endorectal) with functional imaging is the future in assessing the prostate after focal therapy. In a small study, Cirrilo et al. found that the combination of endorectal MRI and PSA was a good method for assessment of recurrence [18] with all the cancers detected when both methods were employed. In a pilot study with nine patients imaged at 6 weeks and 6 months post-HIFU, we found that ADC at 6 weeks was an indicator of subsequent reduction in PSA [19] (Figure 8.5). Kim and colleagues [20] showed that for prediction of local tumor progression after HIFU, a combination of T2W with DW-MRI was more specific (74–78%) although less sensitive than DCE-MRI. Addition of DW-MRI to the conventional T2W images has also been shown to increase the sensitivity and specificity for detecting recurrence following radiotherapy.

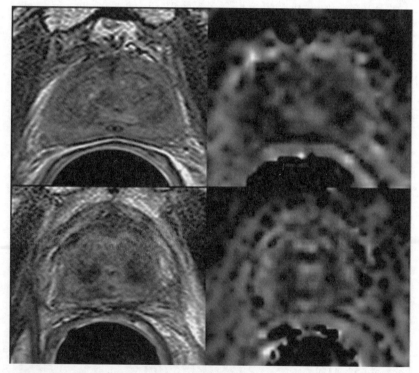

Figure 8.5   Endorectal MRI performed prior (top row) and at 6 weeks post-HIFU (bottom row). T2W transverse images are demonstrated on the left with the corresponding matched ADC map on the right. The T2W images demonstrate a moderate reduction in the tumor volume with an increase in the mean overall ADC of the prostate (more pixels of higher value) after HIFU treatment.

Summary

Diffusion-weighted imaging is becoming increasingly important in the diagnostic armamentarium for prostate cancer. Used in conjunction with T2W imaging, it improves sensitivity and specificity for tumor detection, particularly in the PZ and is showing potential in predicting response and detecting recurrence following locally ablative therapies.

Acknowledgments

We acknowledge the support received for the CRUK and EPSRC Cancer Imaging Centre in association with the MRC and Department of Health (England) grant C1060/A10334. We acknowledge NHS funding to the NIHR Biomedical Research Centre. Sophie Riches is funded by a Personal Award Scheme Researcher Developer Award from the National Institute for Health Research.

References

1. Kirkham AP, et al. How good is MRI at detecting and characterising cancer within the prostate? *Eur Urol* 2006;50(6): 1163–1174.
2. Zelhof B, et al. Correlation of diffusion-weighted magnetic resonance data with cellularity in prostate cancer. *BJUInt* 2009;103(7): 883–888.
3. Kitajima K, et al. High b-value diffusion-weighted imaging in normal and malignant peripheral zone tissue of the prostate: effect of signal-to-noise ratio. *Magn Reson Med Sci* 2008;7(2): 93–99.
4. deSouza NM, et al. A solid reusable endorectal receiver coil for magnetic resonance imaging of the prostate: design, use, and comparison with an inflatable endorectal coil. *J Magn Reson Imaging* 1996; 6(5): 801–804.
5. deSouza NM, et al. Diffusion-weighted magnetic resonance imaging: a potential non-invasive marker of tumor aggressiveness in localized prostate cancer. *Clin Radiol* 2008;63(7): 774–782.
6. deSouza NM, et al. Magnetic resonance imaging in prostate cancer: the value of apparent diffusion coefficients for identifying malignant nodules. *Br J Radiol* 2007;80(950): 90–95.
7. Gibbs P, et al. Comparison of quantitative T2 mapping and diffusion-weighted imaging in the normal and pathologic prostate. *Magn Reson Med* 2001;46(6): 1054–1058.
8. Hosseinzadeh K, Schwarz SD. Endorectal diffusion-weighted imaging in prostate cancer to differentiate malignant and benign peripheral zone tissue. *J Magn Reson Imaging* 2004;20(4): 654–661.
9. Sato C, et al. Differentiation of noncancerous tissue and cancer lesions by apparent diffusion coefficient values in transition and peripheral zones of the prostate. *J Magn Reson Imaging* 2005;21(3): 258–262.

10. Issa B. In vivo measurement of the apparent diffusion coefficient in normal and malignant prostatic tissues using echo-planar imaging. *J Magn Reson Imaging* 2002;16(2): 196–200.
11. Reinsberg SA, et al. Combined use of diffusion-weighted MRI and 1H MR spectroscopy to increase accuracy in prostate cancer detection. *AJR Am J Roentgenol* 2007;188(1): 91–98.
12. Shimofusa R, et al. Diffusion-weighted imaging of prostate cancer. *J Comput Assist Tomogr* 2005; 29(2): 149–153.
13. Morgan VA, et al. Evaluation of the potential of diffusion-weighted imaging in prostate cancer detection. *Acta Radiol* 2007;48(6): 695–703.
14. Lim HK, et al. Prostate cancer: apparent diffusion coefficient map with T2-weighted images for detection—a multireader study. *Radiology* 2009;250(1): 145–151.
15. Haider MA, et al. Combined T2-Weighted and Diffusion-Weighted MRI for Localization of Prostate Cancer. *Am J Roentgenol* 2007;189(2): 323–328.
16. Desouza NM, et al. Magnetic resonance imaging in prostate cancer: the value of apparent diffusion coefficients for identifying malignant nodules. *Br J Radiol* 2007;80(950): 90–95.
17. Mazaheri Y, et al. Prostate tumor volume measurement with combined T2-weighted imaging and diffusion-weighted MR: correlation with pathologic tumor volume. *Radiology* 2009;252(2): 449–457.
18. Cirillo S, et al. Endorectal magnetic resonance imaging and magnetic resonance spectroscopy to monitor the prostate for residual disease or local cancer recurrence after transrectal high-intensity focused ultrasound. *BJU Int* 2008;102(4): 452–458.
19. Chapman A, et al. Evaluation of the prostate after treatment with high-intensity focussed ultrasound (HIFU) therapy using whole prostate diffusion weighted imaging (DWI) analysis. *Proceedings 16th Scientific Meeting, International Society for Magnetic Resonance in Medicine; 2008*, Hawaii.
20. Kim CK, et al. MRI techniques for prediction of local tumor progression after highintensity focusedultrasonic ablation of prostate cancer. *AJR Am J Roentgenol* 2008;190(5): 1180–1186.

CHAPTER 9

The Future of Molecular and Biomolecular Imaging in Prostate Cancer

Michael S. Gee MD PhD and Mukesh G. Harisinghani MD
Section of Abdominal Imaging and Interventional Radiology, Department of Radiology,
Massachusetts General Hospital, Harvard Medical School, Boston, MA, USA

Introduction

Conventionalimaging modalities used to evaluate prostate cancer include transrectal ultrasound (TRUS), computed tomography (CT), and magnetic resonance imaging (MRI) [1]. These imaging technologies all evaluate structural anatomy by exposing the body to energy and resolving intrinsic contrast differences among tissues [2]. TRUS can visualize the prostate gland but cannot reliably discriminate normal from malignant tissue; as such, its role in prostate cancer management is primarily limited to guiding prostate biopsies in patients with suspected disease as well as placement of brachytherapy seeds. MRI is used for primary tumor visualization and detection of locally invasive disease, while CT is primarily used for disease staging through detection of distal disease, including nodal and osseous metastases. In contrast to these traditional anatomic imaging techniques, molecular imaging evaluates changes in cellular physiology and function accompanying disease that are likely to be earlier and more sensitive disease manifestations than anatomically visible lesions. Additionally, molecular imaging seeks to noninvasively evaluate specific molecular pathways in vivo that contribute to the malignant phenotype, and as newer cancer therapies become increasingly molecule-specific, molecular imaging potentially can provide noninvasive determination of patients likely to benefit from treatment as well as early therapy response. These molecular imaging methods are used either alone or in combination with conventional imaging modalities.

Molecular imaging methods

MRI-based imaging techniques

Multiple MRI-based molecular imaging technologies have been developed that can be used in conjunction with conventional MRI to detect prostate tumors. Dynamic contrast-enhanced (DCE) MRI seeks to measure microvascular density and permeability that are characteristically increased in prostate cancer. It involves high temporal resolution T1-weighted imaging sequences obtained immediately following intravenous contrast administration to measure contrast accumulation within tumor blood vessels as well as subsequent contrast passage into the extravascular extracellular space (Chapter 7). The measurements obtained by DCE are mathematically fit into two-compartment pharmacokinetics models to produce wash-in and wash-out kinetics constants. DCE provides a time course of tissue contrast enhancement from which quantitative kinetics parameters can be derived related to prostate cancer, including K_{trans} (volume transfer constant) and k_{ep} (rate constant of exchange between plasma and extracellular and extravascular space)(Figure 9.1).

MR spectroscopy imaging (MRSI) combines conventional MRI anatomic imaging with spectroscopic evaluation of cellular metabolites. In the prostate, the important metabolites are choline and citrate. Choline is an important component of cell membranes, integrated into phospholipid bilayer. Prostate malignancy is hypothesized to lead to increased choline uptake because of increased cell proliferation as well as increased transmembrane signaling. Citrate is a component of the citric acid cycle that normally accumulates within the glandular ducts formed by prostate epithelial cells. Prostate malignancy is thought to lead to decreased citrate levels via increased tumor metabolic activity as well as decreased glandular

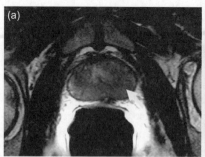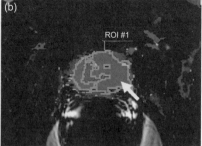

Figure 9.1 Dynamic contrast-enhanced MRI detection of prostate cancer. T2-weighted (a) and DCE MRI K_{trans} maps (b) demonstrate a tumor in the left-peripheral zone that was proven to be prostate cancer by histology. The elevation in K_{trans} exhibited by the tumor is thought to reflect increased vascular permeability and surface area associated with tumor neovascularization. (See Plate 9.1.)

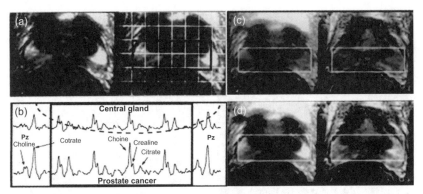

Figure 9.2 MR spectroscopy of prostate cancer. MRI and MR spectroscopy performed on a 48 year old male with an elevated PSA demonstrate a T2 hypointense mass (a; circle) occupying the peripheral zone of the left mid gland with an irregular prostate capsule. Multivoxel MR spectroscopy (b) demonstrates an elevated choline:citrate in multiple voxels (circle) corresponding to the mass. A Gleason grade 9 adenocarcinoma at this location was found at surgery. Images courtesy of Sadhna Verma, MD. (See Plate 9.2.)

differentiation [3] (Figure 9.2). High-resolution three-dimensional quantitative proton spectroscopy can be performed using endorectal surface coils and volumetric spectroscopic sequences.

Diffusion-weighted MR imaging (DW-MRI) is a technique based on detecting changes in the random movement of water molecules that accompany the malignant phenotype. The primary quantitative measure of DW-MRI is the apparent diffusion coefficient (ADC). A number of cancers demonstrate low ADC values, which is thought to reflect reduction in diffusion of water in the intracellular and extracellular compartments. Traditionally, this has been attributed to increased cell density, although other tumor features such as tumor cell organization, high nuclear to cytoplasmic ratio, and tumor cell size are likely to also contribute to the measured ADC [4] (Figure 9.3). One advantage of DW-MRI is its ability to characterize tissue without the need for intravenous contrast (Chapter 8).

Lymphotropic superparamagnetic iron oxide particles (USPIO) consist of a monocrystalline superparamagnetic iron oxide core coated with dextrans to prolong circulation time. These particles, when injected intravenously, are taken up by lymphatic vessels and accumulate within lymph nodes where they are internalized by macrophages. Normal uptake of USPIO in lymph nodes results in magnetic susceptibility effects of iron oxide manifesting as decrease in signal intensity on T2-weighted (T2W) MRI. However, in malignant lymph nodes tumor cells displace normal sinus macrophages leading to reduced USPIO uptake and maintenance of high signal on T2W-MRI. Lymphotropic nanoparticle-enhanced MRI (LN-MRI) provides a way to distinguish malignant and benign lymph nodes during

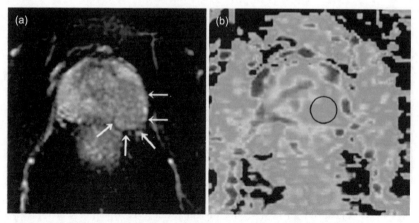

Figure 9.3 MR diffusion-weighted imaging of prostate cancer. T2-weighted (a) and apparent diffusion coefficient (ADC) maps (b) from a 58-year-old male with known prostate cancer demonstrate restricted diffusion (circle) corresponding to the region of the patient's biopsy-proved left-peripheral zone tumor (arrows). (From Tamada T, et al. Apparent diffusion coefficient values in peripheral and transition zones of the prostate: comparison between normal and malignant prostatic tissues and correlation with histologic grade. *JMRI* 2008; **28:**720–726, reproduced with permission of John Wiley & Sons, Inc.) (See Plate 9.3.)

cancer staging, which is often difficult on the basis of size criteria alone. Preliminary studies have also explored the use of USPIO-enhanced MRI to detect primary malignancies on the basis of USPIO accumulation within tumor-infiltrating macrophages.

PET

Positron-emitted tomography (PET) utilizes compounds labeled with positron-emitting radioisotopes as molecular probes [5]. Since tracer accumulation leads to emission of positron pairs at 180° angles to each other, three-dimensional spatial reconstructions of probe localization can be performed. The most commonly used clinical PET probe is the ^{18}F-labeled glucose analog 2-^{18}F-2-deoxy-D-glucose (FDG). This probe is internalized into cells through glucose transporters and phosphorylated; however, the phosphorylated product does not undergo further processing and is retained within cells in proportion to their rate of glycolysis. Many tumor cells are known to have increased glycolytic rates relative to normal cells (known as the Warburg effect), and this association of increased glycolysis with malignancy forms the rationale for using FDG-PET as a method of detecting tumors. Unlike other malignancies, FDG-PET has not demonstrated high accuracy rates for prostate cancer detection. This has been attributed to the relatively indolent growth rate of prostate cancer cells associated with low tumor cell glycolysis, as well as difficulty localizing tumor FDG activity due to urinary tracer excretion. FDG-PET has been shown to have decreased sensitivity for prostate cancer detection compared with CT, as well as reduced accuracy for distinguishing prostate cancer from benign prostate hypertrophy and for detecting prostate cancer recurrence following surgery.

Alternative PET tracers have been developed for prostate cancer detection to overcome the problems associated with FDG. These include ^{11}C-Choline, which is a precursor of phosphatidylcholine, a primary phospholipid component of the cell membrane. ^{11}C-Choline accumulates in proliferating tumor cells undergoing increased cell membrane lipid synthesis and transmembrane signaling, and has been shown in preliminary studies to be superior to FDG-PET for detecting primary prostate malignancies and metastases. The fact that ^{11}C-choline has minimal urinary excretion also makes it favorable for prostate imaging. Prostate-specific membrane antigen (PSMA) is a cell surface protein that is upregulated on prostate cancer cells and is associated with metastasis and a hormone-independent phenotype. An ^{111}In-labeled monoclonal antibody directed against PSMA (capromab pendetide; ProstaScint[®]) has been approved by the FDA for planar scintigraphic imaging; however, its clinical utility is limited due to poor kinetics of tracer accumulation and poor image quality. This has led to the search for other PSMA-specific probes that can be used with either single photon emission computed tomography (SPECT) or PET. 16β-18F-fluoro-5α-dihydrotestosterone (FDHT) is a testosterone analog designed to exhibit increased prostate specificity by localizing to androgen receptors on prostate cancer cells. PET with ^{18}F-Fluorine is also being explored as an alternative to planar scintigraphic imaging with ^{99m}Tc-MDP for detection of bone metastases. Increased uptake of ^{18}F-Fluorine by malignant bone lesions has been demonstrated and thought to be due to local increases in regional blood flow and bone turnover associated with osseous malignancy. Additionally, the increased sensitivity of PET relative to planar scintigraphy or SPECT is likely to provide an additional diagnostic advantage to ^{18}F-Fluorine PET imaging.

Applications

MRS

LN-MRI
A study of 80 patients with resectable prostate cancer (T1–T3) undergoing LN-MRI with USPIO (Feromoxtran-10) compared LNMRI findings histological lymph node sampling. Lack of signal decrease on T2-weighted images following USPIO administration was found to have 91% sensitivity

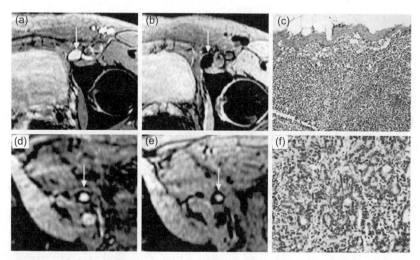

Figure 9.4 LN-MRI detection of prostate cancer metastasis. T2-weighted MRI images of lymph nodes in prostate cancer patients are shown before (a, d) and after (b, e) administration of USPIO, as well as representative histology (c, f) from the lymph nodes after surgical resection. The top row shows a benign lymph node (c) that demonstrates signal loss following USPIO administration (b). The bottom row shows a malignant lymph node (f) that does not accumulate USPIO (e). (From Harisinghani MG, et al. Noninvasive detection of clinically occult lymph-node metastases in prostate cancer. *NEJM* 2003; 348:2491–2499, reproduced with permission. Copyright © 2003 Massachusetts Medical Society, all rights reserved.) (See Plate 9.4.)

and 98% specificity for metastasis on a node-by-node basis (Figure 9.4) [6]. The sensitivity of LN-MRI for lymph node metastasis was statistically increased compared with conventional MRI. Within the subset of smaller lymph node metastases (5–10 mm in short axis diameter) that would be considered normal on conventional CT or MRI, LN-MRI demonstrated 96.4% sensitivity for metastasis. A 2008 study of 60 patients with prostate cancer undergoing LN-MRI also examined whether USPIO could detect the primary prostate malignancy. This study found a statistically signifi-cant association between the magnitude of decrease in prostate gland T2W intensity following USPIO administration and the histological tumor grade, as well as serum PSA elevation, for intermediate and high-grade prostate malignancies [7]. In this case, the USPIO are thought to be taken up by in-filtrating macrophages within the prostate tumor and surrounding stroma.

^{11}C-choline PET

The seminal paper was a 1998 study comparing ^{11}C-choline PET and FDG-PET in 10 patients with prostate cancer, which demonstrated ^{11}C-choline PET to be superior for prostate tumor detection due to high tumor uptake and low urinary excretion [8]. A 2006 study examined ^{11}C-choline PET-CT for detection of primary prostate cancer in 36 patients with known prostate cancer scheduled to undergo radical prostatectomy. ^{11}C-choline PET-CT demonstrated 66% sensitivity and 81% specificity on a sextant basis compared with histologic standard [9]. This high specificity demonstrated in this study was interpreted with caution because of the selected patient population, which consisted of retrospectively enrolled subjects with known histologically proven prostate cancer. In a second study looking at ^{11}C-choline PET in 19 patients with either prostate cancer or benign prostatic hypertrophy, ^{11}C-choline PET exhibited a high false-positive rate for prostate cancer detection, with no significant difference in standard uptake value between within areas of cancer and benign prostatic hypertrophy [10].

^{18}F-FDHT PET

An initial feasibility study of ^{18}F-FDHT PET was performed in 2004 on seven patients with known metastatic prostate cancer [11]. Both ^{18}F-FDHT PET and FDG-PET were performed on each patient, in addition to conventional imaging. A total of 59 bone and soft tissue metastases were identified on conventional imaging, FDG-PET was positive in 97% of the lesions while ^{18}F-FDHT PET was positive in 78% of lesions. A 2005 study evaluating ^{18}F-FDHT-PET imaging of 20 patients with advanced prostate cancer (Figure 9.5) demonstrates a sensitivity of 86% for detection of metastatic lesions identified on conventional imaging [12]. Additionally, 12 patients with detectable disease underwent a second follow-up ^{18}F-FDHT PET 24 hours after initiation of antiandrogen therapy with flutamide. The standard uptake value of lesions on the posttreatment PET was significantly lower compared with the pretreatment value, suggesting that ^{18}F-FDHT PET may be useful for not only assessing tumor susceptibility to androgen ablation therapy, but also monitoring early treatment response.

PSMA-PET

A number of small molecule inhibitors of PSMA have been discovered that have been explored as prostate cancer imaging agents. Their small size leads to more efficient delivery to cancer cells relative to antibody-based probes, as well as a more favorable pharmacokinetic profile for use as diagnostic imaging agents. Multiple studies have demonstrated that these small molecule PSMA inhibitors localize specifically to PSMA-positive prostate tumors by both PET and SPECT imaging methods [13]. Biodistribution studies also demonstrated low tissue background. These promising results suggest that PET imaging of PSMA in humans may not be far away.

[18]F-Fluoride PET

A 1999 study validated the use of ^{18}F-Fluoride PET for detecting osseous metastatic disease [14]. This study compared ^{18}F-Fluoride PET and

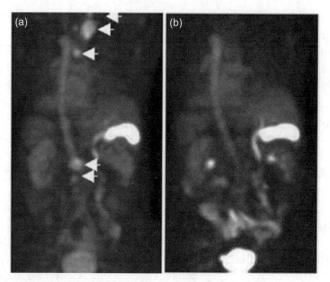

Figure 9.5 FDHT-PET of metastatic prostate cancer. FDHT-PET images of the same patient with metastatic prostate cancer before (a) and 24 hours after (b) hormonal therapy with flutamide demonstrate multiple metastatic mediastinal and retroperitoneal lymph nodes (arrows) whose uptake is abolished following treatment. (From Dehdashti F, et al. Positron tomographic assessment of androgen receptors in prostatic carcinoma. *Eur J Nucl Med Mol Imaging* 2005; 32:344–350, reproduced with permission.)

^{99m}Tc-MDP bone scintigraphy in 44 patients with known prostate, lung, or thyroid carcinoma. Compared with a conventional imaging standard, ^{18}F-Fluoride PET was superior to radionuclide bone scintigraphy for detection of both lytic and blastic bone metastases. A study comparing ^{18}F-Fluoride PET and ^{99m}Tc-MDP bone scintigraphy specifically for detection of bone metastases in prostate cancer performed both examinations the same day in 44 patients with high-risk prostate cancer [15]. Compared with ^{18}F-Fluoride PET-CT reference standard, ^{18}F-Fluoride PET demonstrated 100% sensitivity and 62% specificity for osseous metastases compared with 70% and 57%, respectively for planar bone scintigraphy. ^{18}F-Fluoride PET was more sensitive than both planar bone scintigraphy and multiple field of view SPECT for detection of bone metastases (Figure 9.6).

Conclusions

Molecular imaging will be of increasing importance in the near future as prostate cancer treatments become more molecularly targeted, a trend that has been observed in other urinary tract malignancies. For example, multiple small molecule tyrosine kinase inhibitors (sunitinib, sorafenib)

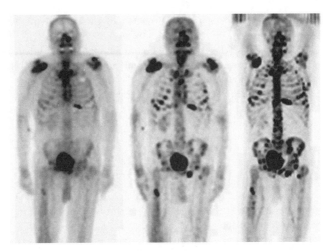

Figure 9.6 ^{18}F-fluoride PET of prostate cancer osseous metastases. Images are from an 82-year-old patient with known metastatic prostate cancer. From left to right: Tc-MDP planar bone scan, Tc-MDP multifield of view SPECT, ^{18}F-fluoride PET. ^{18}F fluoride reveals numerous osseous metastases not seen by Tc-MDP. (Images courtesy of Professor Einat Even-Sapir.)

have recently been introduced into the clinic for treating metastatic renal cell carcinoma. As has been discussed, androgen ablation is already a mainstay of prostate cancer treatment and androgen receptor imaging is a promising diagnostic approach. As our knowledge of prostate cancer signaling pathways expands and more molecularly targeted prostate cancer therapies reach the clinic, effective molecular imaging techniques would be of tremendous benefit as a screen for drug and ablative treatment susceptibility, an aid in optimizing individual patient therapy, and as an early marker of efficacy and refractoriness.

References

1. Kelloff GJ, et al. Challenges in clinical prostate cancer: role of imaging. AJR *Am J Roentgenol* 2009;192: 1455–1470.
2. Weissleder R, Ntziachristos V: Shedding light onto live molecular targets. *Nat Med* 2003;9: 123–128.
3. Kurhanewicz J, et al: Three-dimensional H-1 MR spectroscopic imaging of the in situ human prostate with high (0.24–0.7-cm3) spatial resolution. *Radiology* 1996;198: 795–805.
4. Tamada T, et al: Apparent diffusion coefficient values in peripheral and transition zones of the prostate: comparison between normal and malignant prostatic tissues and correlation with histologic grade. *JMRI* 2008;28: 720–726.
5. Phelps ME. Inaugural article: positron emission tomography provides molecular imaging of biological processes. *PNAS-USA* 2000;97: 9226–9233.

6. Harisinghani MG, et al: Noninvasive detection of clinically occult lymph-node metastases in prostate cancer. *NEJM* 2003;348: 2491–2499.

7. Li CS, et al: Enhancement characteristics of ultrasmall superparamagnetic iron oxide particle within the prostate gland in patients with primary prostate cancer. *J Comput Assist Tomogr* 2008;32: 523–528.

8. Hara T, et al. PET imaging of prostate cancer using carbon-11-choline. *J Nucl Med* 1998;39: 990–995.

9. Farsad M, et al: Detection and localization of prostate cancer: correlation of (11)C-choline PET/CT with histopathologic step-section analysis. *J Nucl Med* 2005;46: 1642–1649.

10. Sutinen E, et al. Kinetics of [(11)C]choline uptake in prostate cancer: a PET study. *Eur J Nucl Med Mol Imaging* 2004;31: 317–324.

11. Larson SM, et al. Tumor localization of 16beta-18F-fluoro-5alpha-dihydro-testosterone versus 18F-FDG in patients with progressive, metastatic prostate cancer. *J Nucl Med* 2004;45: 366–373.

12. Dehdashti F, et al. Positron tomographic assessment of androgen receptors in prostatic carcinoma. *Eur J Nucl Med Mol Imaging* 2005;32: 344–350.

13. Foss CA, et al. Radiolabeled small-molecule ligands for prostate-specific membrane antigen: in vivo imaging in experimental models of prostate cancer. *Clin Cancer Res* 2005;11: 4022–4028.

14. Schirrmeister H, et al. Sensitivity in detecting osseous lesions depends on anatomic localization: planar bone scintigraphy versus 18F PET. *J Nucl Med* 1999;40: 1623–1629.

15. Even-Sapir E, et al. The detection of bone metastases in patients with high-risk prostate cancer: 99mTc-MDP Planar bone scintigraphy, single- and multi-field-of-view SPECT, 18F-fluoride PET, and 18F-fluoride PET/CT. *J Nucl Med* 2006;47: 287–297.

SECTION III

How can we create discrete tissue necrosis?

CHAPTER 10

Energies for Focal Ablation: Cyroablation

John F. Ward MD FACS

Department of Urology, The University of Texas, MD Anderson Cancer Center, Houston, TX, USA

Introduction

Early cryoablative techniques employed a brine (water + salt) cryogen to treat numerous conditions, including headaches and neuralgia. At a concentration of 23.3%, the freezing point of sodium chloride brine is −21°C and that of calcium chloride brine is −40°C. While these temperatures are capable of causing cell injury and death, rapid warming of the brine solution and difficulty in applying these solutions to internally located structures confounded reliable and repeatable tissue targeting and destruction. Between 1845 and 1851, Dr. James Arnott of Brighton, England, used brine solutions to treat cervical and breast tumors reporting both tumor shrinkage and a significant decrease in pain [1]. He later designed an apparatus for the application of cold, which was shown at the Great Exhibition in London in 1851. However, the device was cumbersome to use, had little freezing capability, and found little clinical applicability.

Following World War II, Irving Cooper (a physician) and Arnold Lee (an engineer) collaborated to build a cryosurgical probe that would eventually be the prototype for all subsequent cryosurgical probes. Their design consisted of three long concentric tubes that allowed for closed-loop circulation of a liquid cryogen [2]. The liquefied cryogen was forced at pressure through the inner tube to the tip of the probe, while the space between the inner tube and the middle tube provided a path for the return of the expanded, warmed gaseous form of the cryogen. The third space, between the outer tube and the middle tube, was vacuum insulated with a radiative shield to prevent countercurrent heat exchange. While many cryogens were examined (oxygen, nitrous oxide, carbon dioxide, argon, ethyl chloride, fluorinated hydrocarbons), liquid nitrogen became the cryogen of

Focal Therapy in Prostate Cancer, First Edition. Edited by Hashim U Ahmed, Manit Arya, Peter Carroll and Mark Emberton.

choice because it is nonflammable, nonexplosive, nontoxic, readily abundant, and inexpensive.

Dr. Cooper introduced these probes for cryogenic surgery of parenchymal lesions through a paper in the *New England Journal of Medicine* in 1966 [3]. Urologists quickly saw the potential for targeting the prostate with this new instrument and were at the forefront of this renewed interest in cryoablative techniques, with one of the first applications being to treat benign prostatic hyperplasia and subsequently to treat prostate cancer via an open-perineal approach. A closed, transperineal approach with a single cryoprobe that was digitally guided and repositioned as necessary during the procedure to freeze the palpable prostate was introduced in 1974 [4]. At that time, the complications of the closed, transperineal approach were felt to be less debilitating than those associated with a radical prostatectomy, but the approach was poorly accepted because of the difficulty in monitoring cryoprobe placement and ice-ball formation.

The "second generation" of prostate cryoablation began in 1988 when Dr. Onik and colleagues introduced transrectal ultrasound as a real-time guide for monitoring cryotherapy [5]. Again, urologists quickly adopted the procedure for transrectal monitoring of prostate ice formation, and ultrasound gained widespread use through the 1990s when a multiple cryoprobe system was introduced and then a urethral warmer device, which consisted of a closed double-lumen catheter through which heated saline (38–42°C) was continuously circulated with a water pump. Unfortunately, just as the number of patients being treated with prostate cryoablation began to increase, the urethral warmer device produced by Cryomedical Sciences (Kennesaw, GA) was taken off the market for a brief time by the Food and Drug Administration (FDA) to complete a safety and efficacy evaluation. During this time, many serious complications occurred and acceptance of cryotherapy for the treatment of localized prostate cancer met resistance.

The "third generation" of cryoablation originated in 2001 with the introduction of a cryotherapy system based on argon gas cryogen rather than liquid nitrogen. The rapid expansion of argon gas through a small opening within the tip of the cryoprobe cools the tip to −150°C and can be quickly exchanged with helium to induce an active thawing phase (Figure 10.1). This is due to the Joule–Thomson effect in which a temperature change occurs when a gas is forced through a valve and allowed to undergo free expansion in a vacuum.

At room temperature, all gases except hydrogen, helium, and neon cool upon expansion. Modern cryosystems can use the same Joule–Thomson effect to achieve both cooling with argon gas and tissue warming with helium gas. Since gas can be more easily circulated through a small tube, the cryoprobes (still using the same Cooper design) were reduced in diameter from 3 mm (which required a tissue dilator to place the blunt tipped probe)

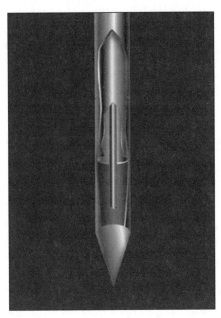

Figure 10.1   Engineering drawing of gas-driven cryoprobe. Use of gas rather than liquid allowed for smaller needle diameter and subsequently direct prostate access. The Joule–Thomson effect allows the single cryoprobe to both cool and warm the tissue by using Argon and Helium gasses, respectively. (See Plate 10.1.)

to the current 1.5-mm (17-gauge) cryoprobes; these cryoprobes have a sharp, pointed design and can be directly inserted into the prostate without tissue dilation using the transperineal approach.

The development of the third generation of cryoablation technology has allowed for the creation of smaller ice zones thereby conforming the ice ball to the individual's unique prostate configuration through pretreatment planning and the placement of multiple cryoprobes. Recently, this concept has been further refined with the introduction of variable ice probes, which allow the user to not only configure the diameter of the ice formation but also its length (Figure 10.2). This evolution of technology has only now allowed us to consider performing organ-preserving prostate cryoablation. The confluence of imaging through transrectal ultrasound, a safe and efficacious urethral warmer, and the reduced needle size all allow variable ice formation that is accurately applied, predictable, and monitored to make organ-preserving therapy possible.

Cryobiology

Study of the mechanism of tissue injury (cryobiology) parallels the ebb and flow of clinical practice in cryosurgery, although a much larger body of

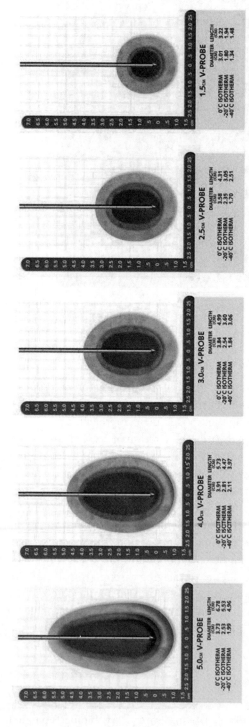

Figure 10.2 Isotherms and ice ball dimensions for cryoprobe. Current technology allows cryoprobes to be individually adjusted to alter the ice ball length and shape. Through careful placement of cryoprobes and adjustment of the ice ball formations, the targeted area for destruction can be selectively treated using these instruments.

work exists for cells frozen in the presence of cryoprotective agents for cryopreservation purposes. Understanding the multiplicity of potential mechanisms of injury and death is important to achieve the desired targeted effect with subtotal prostate cryoablation.

Direct cellular injury is the best known and most described mechanism of cellular injury in cryobiology. Direct cellular injury depends on thermal history but occurs through two physical changes: dehydration and ice crystal formation. At low cooling rates, osmotic dehydration occurs as the solute concentration outside the cell increases. This dehydration in turn draws water from the cell, resulting in damage to the enzymatic machinery and a destabilized cell membrane. Alternatively, at rapid cooling rates, the water is trapped inside the cell and results in a super cooling of the cytoplasm and ultimately ice crystal formation that damages both organelles and membranes. These two different mechanisms of direct cell injury result in an inverse curve of cell viability with low viability at extremely rapid and extremely slow cooling rates but high viability at cooling rates between these extremes.

In patients, the cooling and thawing rates are often highly nonlinear and vary throughout the prostate because of tissue heterogeneity and nonuniform heat sinks provided by both vascular structures (dorsal vein complex, neurovascular bundles, prostatic arterioles) and the urethral warmer. However, in general, a lower temperature increases the probability of cell death. Using various prostate cancer cell lines, it has been shown that a decrease in cell viability occurs from about 35% at −20°C to 5% at −40°C. When these lethal end temperatures are achieved, the cooling rate appears to have much less impact on cell viability.

For organ-preserving prostate cryotherapy, monitoring the temperature at the targeted site of destruction is therefore at least as important as monitoring temperatures at vital structures intended for preservation to assure a "lethal" end temperature is achieved. This will theoretically allow slower rates of freezing if necessary to provide the structural preservation desired without compromising oncologic outcome.

Vascular injury is a second but less predictable mechanism by which tissue is both destroyed and preserved with prostate cryoablation. The fact that freezing preferentially destroys the microvasculature over larger blood vessels suggests that cryoinjury affects nutrient and oxygen delivery and may induce necrosis beyond the region of lethal ice formation. This vascular injury has the potential to expand the area of destroyed tissue beyond the target zone. As this effect is less predictable, vascular injury is not used in planning the treatment zone with subtotal prostate cryoablation but may be the source of morbidity related to tissue injury outside the zone of lethal ice.

Direct cellular injury occurs during the freeze portion of cryoablation, and vascular injury is believed to be critical to tissue damage that occurs during the thawing portion of the procedure. Perivascular cellular dehydration results in vessel distention and engorgement with direct endothelial cell injury, exposure of the underlying thrombogenic connective tissue, and propagation of thrombus formation. This perivascular cellular dehydration could explain why anticoagulation has been found to limit tissue injury after freezing. Additionally, vasoactive factors released during thawing allow for vessel dilatation and hyperperfusion with high oxygen delivery purported to cause peroxidation of the lipids in the membrane and subsequent free-radical formation. Thawing injuries have also been shown to be secondary to neutrophil recruitment, which is secondary to cellular debris and necrosis.

Researchers of cryobiology have also investigated other mechanisms of response to hypothermia that may play a role in the future of subtotal prostate cryoablation. Hypothermia is a cellular stressor that can induce selective gene expression such as interleukin-8, fibroblast growth factor, and vascular endothelial growth factors. These selective gene expressions may offer both therapeutic targets to either enhance tumor cell destruction or conversely provide a means of preserving normal tissues. Subtotal prostate cryoablation may also have a role as part of treatment-induced immunotherapy for both localized small, and yet undetected carcinomas within the prostate as well as the potential means of inducing a broader immune response [6].

Clinical reports of organ-preserving prostate cryoablation

Three clinical trials of subtotal prostate cryoablation have been reported [7–9]. As with any current strategy for organ-preserving prostate cancer ablative therapy, these series vary in their eligibility criteria and in the amount of tissue targeted for destruction and preservation (Table 10.1) [10].

Lambert et al. carried out hemiablative treatment in 25 men with unilaterally positive prostate biopsy (12 cores) in which with less than 10% tumor volume was present in one or two contiguous biopsy cores [7]. At diagnosis, 24 were potent with 4 using phosphodiesterase-5 inhibitors at the time of treatment. The mean age was 69 years (range 61–78) with a median follow-up of 28 months. Potency was preserved postoperatively in 17 patients (71%), with 7 using phosphodiesterase-5 inhibitors. There was no urinary incontinence, rectal pain, perineal discomfort, or fistula formation. Freedom from biochemical recurrence, defined by ASTRO

Table 10.1 Reports of clinical trials of organ-preserving prostate cryoablation. (Reproduced with permission from Polascik TJ, Mouraviev V. Focal therapy for prostate cancer. *Curr Opin Urol* 2008;18: 269–274.)

Reference	Number of patients	Number of Biopsy cores	Median follow up (months)	Cryounit	bDFS[a] (%)	PSA cutoff	Biopsy-proven recurrence	Potency preserved
Unilateral cryoablation of unilateral lesions								
Lambert et al. [7] (3.5-year data)	25	12	28	SeedNet[a]	84 88	<50% nadir nadir + 2	12% 8% untreated lobe; 4% treated lobe;	71%
Bahn et al. [8] (5-year data)[b]	31	6–12	70	Cryocare[c]	93	ASTRO[d]	4% untreated lobe	88.9% total; 48.1% fully recovered, 40.8% medically assisted
Focal cryoablation of unifocal lesion Onik [9] (6-year data)	21	7–8	50 (mean)	Cryocare	96 95	Negative Bx ASTRO	0 [in one (5%) case cancer was found on MRIS in untreated lobe]	80%

Bx, biopsy; bDFS, biochemical disease-free survival; PSA, prostate-specific antigen; MRIS, MRI spectroscopy.
[a] SeedNet, Galil Medical, Plymouth Meeting, Pennsylvania, USA
[b] Results of two-center clinical trail.
[c] Cryocare, Endocare, Irvine, California, USA.
[d] American Society for Therapeutic Radiology and Oncology (ASTRO) definition; three subsequent PSA rises [32.]
Reproduced from Future Oncol. (2007) 3(5): 569–574 with permission of Future Medicine Ltd.

(American Society of Therapeutic Radiology and Oncology)-Phoenix criteria—serum prostate specific antigen (PSA) nadir + 2 ng/mL—was achieved in 21 (88%). Seven patients had prostate biopsy following hemiablation, with two men positive on the contralateral side and one recurrence on the treated side; all had a Gleason score of 6 with tumor volumes of less than 5%. All three men with recurrences underwent a second cryotherapy treatment and were rendered biochemically disease-free at the time of the report. This study highlights the difficult problem of treatment based on a random sampling of the prostate through the core biopsy process and the problem of very high rate of contralateral prostate cancer when undertaking unilateral ablation [11]. Nonetheless, it does demonstrate the safety and effectiveness of repeat cryoablations for persistent disease or undetected contralateral disease, an important concept when considering long-term management of patients undergoing an organ-preserving technique.

Bahn et al. attempted to address the problem of random sampling of the prostate by requiring a Doppler transrectal ultrasound with biopsy of all suspicious areas prior to prostate hemiablation in 31 men [8]. At 70 months follow-up, 93% were biochemically free of disease (defined by ASTRO criteria—three consecutive PSA increases) with 96% (24/25) having no cancer on posttreatment biopsy; the single patient with persistent cancer at the contralateral apex was retreated with full-gland cryotherapy. Potency was preserved in 89% (24/27) of men, with 11 requiring phosphodiesterase-5 inhibitors. This study highlights the importance of patient selection for subtotal prostate gland therapy; developing technologies such as Doppler ultrasound, contrast-enhanced ultrasound, tissue characterization ultrasound (e.g., Histoscanning®), elastography, or multiparametric magnetic resonance imaging will help to detect cancers suitable for subtotal ablation with the eventual goal of guiding ablation in real time.

In a study by Onik et al., 48 men with unilateral prostate cancer predominantly demonstrated on three-dimensional transperineal template mapping biopsy received targeted focal cryotherapy to the lobe which was positive. Some of these men had only transrectal diagnostic biopsies prior to hemiablative cryotherapy [9] Follow-up ranged from 2 years to 10 years with a mean of 4.5 years; 45 (94%) had stable PSAs as defined by ASTRO criteria. Eight percent (4/48) had positive histology in the contralateral side and underwent redo-cryotherapy to the whole prostate. None had persistent disease in the treated side. Potency with this approach was maintained in 90% (36/40). Onik et al. presented encouraging results of 21 patients who had reached 6-year follow-up (part of the same cohort) in a different publication (Table 10.1) [12].

This study highlights the debate regarding the amount of prostate tissue that should be ablated to achieve best oncologic efficacy versus the

Table 10.2 Organ-preserving prostate ablation templates and nomenclature. (Modified from Ward JF, Jones JS. Classification system: organ preserving treatment for prostate cancer. *Urology* 2010.)

Name	Schematic description	Narrative description
Nerve-sparing prostate ablation (unilateral or bilateral)		Destruction of all prostatic tissue excepting the posterior lateral on one or both sides of the prostate
Hemiablation of the prostate		Destruction of all prostate tissue within lateralized hemisphere
Anterior hockey stick (3/4 ablation)		Hemiablation of the prostate PLUS anterior contralateral region
Posterior hockey stick (3/4 ablation)		Hemiablation of the prostate PLUS posterior contralateral region
Targeted focal therapy		Very limited destruction of prostate tissue isolated to the area of known tumor. Requires detailed prostate-mapping biopsy
Zonal ablation		Destruction of sector (anterior or posterior sextant) containing prostate cancer after extended prostate biopsy using spatial-targeting device

amount that can be ablated and still maintain the high potency and continence rates for which this subtotal approach is being applied. As the field of organ-preserving prostate cancer treatments advances, reporting on the ablative template applied will be important for our communication about and understanding of these two competing outcomes. A recommended nomenclature for discussing organ-preserving templates is presented by Ward and Jones (Table 10.2) [13].

Conclusions

Cryoablation is an effective means of tissue destruction that is capable of precise control. The current technology allows this ablative energy to be applied in a number of different configurations to achieve varying degrees of tissue destruction and preservation. The FDA has approved this technology for tissue destruction, and cryoablation is available for immediate use. A few retrospective studies have been conducted with which are somewhat limited by patient numbers, incomplete reporting and lack of validated tools to measure outcomes. Nonetheless, these early reports suggest multiple goals of functional preservation and cancer control can be achieved simultaneously with an outpatient procedure. Ongoing prospective trials with validated quality-of-life instruments and longer follow-up are still needed.

References

1. Arnott J. Practical illustrations of the remedial efficacy of a very low or anaesthetic temperature. I. In Cancer. *Lancet* 1850;2: 257–259.
2. Cooper IS, Lee AS. Cryostatic congelation: a system for producing a limited, controlled region of cooling or freezing of biologic tissues. *J Nerv Ment Dis* 1961;133: 259–263.
3. Cooper IS, Hirose T. Application of cryogenic surgery to resection of parenchymal organs. *NEJM* 1966;274: 15–18.
4. Megalli MR, et al. Closed perineal cryosurgery in prostatic cancer. New probe and technique. *Urology* 1974;4: 220–222.
5. Onik G, et al. US characteristics of frozen prostate. *Radiology* 1988;168: 629–631.
6. den Brok MH, et al. Efficient loading of dendritic cells following cryo and radiofrequency ablation in combination with immune modulation induces anti-tumour immunity. *BJC* 2006;95: 896–905.
7. Lambert EH, et al. Focal cryosurgery: encouraging health outcomes for unifocal prostate cancer. *Urology* 2007;69: 1117–1120.
8. Bahn DK, et al. Focal Prostate Cryoablation: Initial Results Show Cancer Control and Potency Preservation. *J Endourology* 2006;20: 688–692.

9. Onik G, et al. The "male lumpectomy": focal therapy for prostate cancer using cryoablation results in 48 patients with at least 2-year follow-up. *Urol Oncol* 2008;26: 500–505.

10. Polascik TJ, Mouraviev V. Focal therapy for prostate cancer. *Curr Opin Urol* 2008;18: 269–274.

11. Ward JF, et al. Cancer ablation with regional templates applied to prostatectomy specimens from men who were eligible for focal therapy. *BJUI* 2009.

12. Onik G. The male lumpectomy: rationale for a cancer targeted approach for prostate cryoablation. A review. *Technol Cancer Res Treat* 2004;3: 365–370.

13. Ward JF, Jones JS. Classification System: Organ Preserving Treatment for Prostate Cancer. *Urology* 2010;75(6): pp. 1258–1260.

CHAPTER 11

Focal Salvage Cryoablation in Recurrent Prostate Cancer

Katsuto Shinohara MD

Department of Urology and Radiation Oncology, University of California, San Francisco, San Francisco, CA, USA

Introduction

Radiation is a common form of therapy for patients with newly diagnosed localized prostate cancer. Despite modifications of delivering radiation to the gland, such as intensity modulation, three-dimensional conformal, and computer-assisted seed implantation, a significant number of patients will have a rise in their serum prostate specific antigen (PSA) value in the years after radiation signifying biochemical failure. Approximately, one-third of patients with biochemical failure will have local recurrence [1]. If a local recurrence is detected early, salvage therapy can be initiated. Recent advances in technology and the technique of salvage cryosurgery has led to the ability to eradicate these tumors. However, complications are common after such procedures with incontinence resulting in as high as 72–95% of patients after whole-gland cryotherapy [2]. While newer generation cryosurgery systems have improved outcomes, morbidity remains high (Table 11.1).

Partial cryoablation of the prostate has been explored in the primary treatment setting in an attempt to reduce the morbidity while maintaining oncologic control. Indeed, in this setting and in carefully selected men with unilateral disease, biochemical disease-free rates (BDFS) of 84–95% can be achieved. In addition, surveillance biopsies show low rates of residual carcinoma. Overall, complication rates are low with potency maintained in 68–80%. Thus, partial cryoablation of prostate in carefully selected patients seems to preserve oncologic control with lower rates of morbidity compared to whole-gland ablation in the primary setting. Focus is now turning on men who have had previous radiation therapy to evaluate

---

Focal Therapy in Prostate Cancer, First Edition. Edited by Hashim U Ahmed, Manit Arya, Peter Carroll and Mark Emberton.

Table 11.1 Published complication rates associated with whole-gland salvage cryoablation.

Author	Year	Number of patients	Cryo system generation	Incontinence (%)	Fistula (%)	Urinary obstruction (%)	Pelvic pain (%)
Pisters et al. [3]	1997	150	1st	73	1	67	8
De la Taille et al. [4]	2000	43	2nd	9	0	5	26
Chin et al. [5]	2001	118	2nd	33.3	3.3	8.5	n/a
Ghafar et al. [6]	2001	38	3rd	7.9	0	0	39.5
Bahn et al. [7]	2003	59	2nd	8	3.4	N/A	N/A
Nq et al. [8]	2007	187	3rd	40	2	21	14
Ismail et al. [9]	2007	100	3rd	13	1	4	N/A
Pisters et al. [10]	2008	279	2nd/3rd	4.4	1.2	3.2	N/A

whether such positive returns on morbidity can be seen in this difficult group of men without significantly compromising cancer control [11,12].

Preoperative evaluation and patient selection

PSA

If the PSA should rise in the irradiated patient, the optimal time for intervention is unclear. Most radiation oncologists feel that the PSA can fluctuate within the first few years. A temporary PSA rise after brachytherapy is commonly seen around 20 months after therapy. Such a "bounce" phenomenon can be found following brachytherapy as well as external beam radiation. When considering salvage therapy, the clinician needs to take into account other variables, such as preexisting medical conditions, age, and patient preference. If the PSA should rise above the nadir level consistently, performing a biopsy of the prostate is reasonable. However, a PSA more than 10 ng/mL at the time of diagnosis of local recurrence and a PSA doubling time (PSADT) of less than 16 months will have a poor prognosis after salvage cryosurgery [13]. If PSADT is less than 6 months, there is a significantly higher risk of metastases even if local disease is confirmed by biopsy due to the presence of micrometastatic disease undetected by conventional imaging.

Prostate biopsy

If a biopsy is undertaken, multiple cores should be obtained, and the pathologists need to be informed that the patient has had previous radiation. Benign glands affected by radiation can mimic cancerous glands and special staining, with high molecular weight keratin, may be necessary to make a correct diagnosis. Radiation therapy may not eradicate cancer immediately, and malignant glands may remain as they undergo apoptosis slowly. Such severely affected cancer cells may remain in the prostate as long as 36 months after radiotherapy. Therefore, an expert reading of the postradiation biopsy specimen is essential. As with biopsies in the treatment-naive gland, there are no definite guidelines as to how many cores should be obtained. In order to map out cancer location for consideration of focal ablation, an extended saturation sampling scheme is needed at the very least. Many have advocated template mapping biopsies as this avoids the rectal mucosa and gives precise cancer location to deliver focal therapy. Men who are found to have cancer localized to only one lobe are ideal for focal salvage cryoablation, although the concept of index lesion ablation may also hold merit in the focal salvage setting.

In addition to biopsy of the prostate gland, the seminal vesicles (SV) should also be targeted on each side in this patient group. After radiation therapy, cancer invading the SV may appear normal on imaging. The incidence of SV involvement in men with a rising PSA after radiation and with locally recurrent disease is much higher than the nonirradiated patient; salvage radical prostatectomy series reveal SV involvement as high as 42% [14].

Local recurrence of prostate cancer after radiation appears to be related to tumor burden. A large focus of tumor has a higher risk of incomplete eradication by radiation. Prostate cancer is known for its multifocality, but there is some data to suggest that patterns of local recurrence after radiation therapy can be unifocal or at least clinically significant unifocal disease. The assumption is that small foci in the prostate will be successfully treated by radiation but not necessarily a large index lesion, which is responsible for metastases [15,16]. Therefore, after radiotherapy, unifocal disease is more likely to be found (Figure 11.2). There may be a role for MRI in localization of prostate cancer, but such imaging modalities are unlikely to detect lesions smaller than 0.2 mL in size or Gleason pattern 3 or below [17]. Therefore, we rely on biopsy to localize the cancer, but due to the random and systematic errors associated with transrectal ultrasound-guided biopsies, this can also be imprecise. Further investigation to better validate MR-imaging and biopsy techniques, such as transperineal mapping biopsy [18], to accurately predict the location of recurrence is needed to select the ideal candidate and treatment planning for partial salvage cryoablation.

Metastatic work-up

If a prostate biopsy reveals recurrent disease in the gland, a metastatic evaluation should be performed. The work-up should include a CT-scan of the abdomen and pelvis as well as a radioisotope bone scan. There may be a role in performing an open or laparoscopic pelvic lymph node dissection.

The lymph node positivity rate from salvage radical prostatectomy ranges between 11% and 40%.

Other factors

Prostate size is less of a problem with irradiated patients since their prostate is significantly smaller after radiotherapy. However, patients with a prior history of prostate surgery for benign disease, such as transurethral resection of prostate, should be carefully counseled as such men are at increased risk for urethral necrosis leading to sloughing and incontinence.

Operative technique

During salvage cryoablation, the prostate is generally found to be atrophic, fibrous, and hard. Therefore, smaller 17-gauge probes such as the SeedNet system (Galil Medical Inc., Plymouth Meeting, PA) are preferable. Under general or regional anesthesia in the lithotomy position, a council-tipped catheter is placed in the bladder. Under transrectal ultrasound guidance 2–4 cryoprobes are placed percutaneously through the perineum into the lobe with recurrent carcinoma. The exact number depends on the size of the gland and the area to be ablated (Figure 11.1). Temperature probes are placed in Denonvilliers' fascia in the treating side, the apex, the external sphincter, and the neurovascular bundle ipsilateral to the site of disease recurrence. After placement of all probes, the council-tip catheter should be exchanged for a urethral warming device by means of a guide-wire. Warmed normal saline (43°C) is circulated through the urethral warming device and two freeze-thaw cycles are routinely performed. In the case of a larger prostate gland in which the apex is not completely frozen by the initial freezing cycle, the cryoprobes are slightly withdrawn toward the apex and additional freeze-thaw cycles are carried out. Each freezing cycle

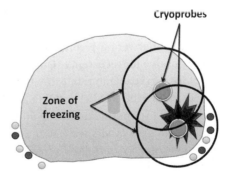

Figure 11.1 Diagram to show typical probe placement in relation to cancer location in focal salvage cryoablation.

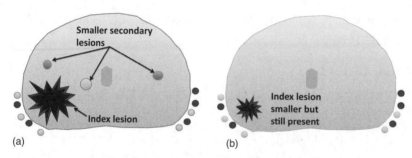

Figure 11.2 Theoretical explanation of prostate cancer distribution in pre- and postradiation therapy. (a) Multiple foci of cancer are present in the prostate with one large index tumor prior to radiation therapy. (b) After radiation therapy, smaller cancer foci are eradicated, but the index lesion is not completely eradicated.

is continued until all temperature probes (except the one at the external sphincter) register at or below −20°C. Patients are usually discharged on the day of the procedure with an indwelling catheter remaining in place for 2–5 days.

Oncological effect

Only one series has so far been published from the University of California San Francisco. Twenty-seven men met the inclusion criteria, of which 24 had greater than 6-months follow-up (Table 11.2). There were no intraoperative or cancer-related deaths. The mean age was 71 years. Salvage treatment was required a mean of 6 years after primary radiotherapy. Primary therapy consisted of external beam radiation alone in 14 men; 10 received brachytherapy in the form of either permanent seed implantation or high dose rate (HDR) brachytherapy; 3 had been treated with salvage HDR after initial local recurrence following external beam radiation; 5 were on some form of hormone ablation therapy, and 1 was hormone refractory at the time of focal salvage therapy. Seventeen men underwent TRUS biopsy 1 year after focal cryoablation with an encouraging 82% (14/17) having no residual carcinoma. Three underwent a second biopsy on further follow-up, of which none were positive for recurrence. One had viable carcinoma ipsilateral to the side of focal cryoablation, but the disease was in the SV, which was not targeted during the focal cryoablation. This same patient also had recurrent disease in the contralateral lobe and was subsequently started on hormone ablation. Two others were found to have viable cancer in the contralateral lobe and SV on follow-up biopsy. No patient had residual cancer in the treated area.

BDFS as defined by the previous definition by American Society for Therapeutic Radiation and Oncology (ASTRO) was 89%, 67%, and

Table 11.2 Characteristics and outcomes of partial salvage cryoablation patients.

N	Total	27
	>6 mos f/u	24
Age		71.0 (58–86)
*Gleason grade before RT	6	2
	7	12
	≥8	10
RT treatment	EBRT	14
	EBRT + Brachy/HDR	10
	Salvage HDR	3
Gland size (mL)		17 (6–29)
Pre-cryo PSA		3.3 (0.28–8.96)
Time to salvage therapy (years)		6 ± 3
Follow-up biopsy	Carcinoma	3/17 (patients)
Complications	Incontinence	1
	Urethral stricture	1
	Urethral ulcer	1
Outcomes	Metastatic disease	3

Brachy, brachytherapy; EBRT, external beam radiotherapy; HDR, high dose rate brachytherapy; RT, radiotherapy)
*Three patients: grade unknown.

50% at 1, 2, and 3 years, respectively. Using the new ASTRO-Phoenix definition, 89%, 79%, and 79% of men were free of biochemical recurrence at 1, 2, and 3 years, respectively [15]. All failures by the ASTRO definition had PSADT < 12 months. Conversely, 1/11 patients without biochemical failure by the ASTRO definition also had a PSADT < 12 months.

Complications

One patient developed mild stress urinary incontinence requiring the use of daily pads. Another patient developed a urethral stricture in the fossa navicularis requiring dilation. One patient developed an ulcer in the prostatic urethra just proximal to the verumontanum after cryoablation; he was managed using a suprapubic catheter with symptomatic resolution occurring after 6 months with cavity formation. Another patient had rectal pain, which resolved by 3 months. Of five men with available potency follow-up data in the form of the International Index of Erectile Function-5 questionnaire, two maintained potency, while three were impotent after treatment.

Conclusions

Given the radiation changes that are inevitably present as well as the advanced age and comorbidities of most patients who have failed primary prostate cancer therapy, a minimally invasive therapy that retains acceptable oncologic control with a lower rate of side effects may be possible with focal cryoablation. Indeed, in properly selected patients with unilateral foci of recurrent adenocarcinoma of the prostate BDFS of 50–79% can be achieved at 3 years; the differing cancer control outcomes reflecting the differences in defining BDFS. These rates are similar to BDFS seen in salvage therapy for prostate cancer.

It is difficult to draw definitive conclusions about the complication rate after focal salvage cryoablation given the small numbers and limited data. Certainly, a 7% incontinence rate and no fistulae are encouraging. One patient developed partial necrosis of the prostatic urethra, which resulted in a cavity formation in the prostate. Even using a urethral warming device, only a portion of the urethra that directly touches the warming catheters membrane can be protected. With a relatively rigid urethral warmer, the floor of the urethra just proximal to the verumontanum is still not completely protected by the urethral warmer, and careful placement of the probes is necessary. By the nature of the patient population treated after failed radiation therapy, alongside age, comorbidities, and the use of prior or current androgen ablation therapy, men generally have moderate-to-severe erectile dysfunction at baseline, so preservation of potency is likely to be difficult to evaluate and expected to be low as a result.

In patients with a unilateral focus of recurrent prostate adenocarcinoma after radiation therapy, acceptable oncologic control can be achieved with minimal morbidity. However, focal cryoablation of the prostate requires careful patient selection as the main problem with this group of men is the presence of microscopic metastatic disease at time of therapy not detected using conventional radioisotope or cross-sectional imaging.

References

1. Shipley WU, et al. Radiation therapy for clinically localized prostate cancer: a multi-institutional pooled analysis. *JAMA* 1999;281: 1598–1604.
2. Nguyen PL, et al. Patient selection, cancer control, and complications after salvage local therapy for postradiation prostate-specific antigen failure: a systematic review of the literature. *Cancer* 2007;110(7): 1417–1428.
3. Pisters LL, et al. The efficacy and complications of salvage cryotherapy of the prostate. *J Urol* 1997;157: 921–925.
4. de la Taille A, et al. Salvage cryotherapy for recurrent prostate cancer after radiation therapy: the Columbia experience. *Urology* 2000;55: 79–84.

5. Chin JL, et al. Results of salvage cryoablation of the prostate after radiation: identifying predictors of treatment failure and complications. *J Urol* 2001;165: 1937–1941.

6. Ghafar MA, et al. Salvage cryotherapy using an argon based system for locally recurrent prostate cancer after radiation therapy: the Columbia experience. *J Urol* 2001;166: 1333–1337; discussion 1337–1338.

7. Bahn DK, et al. Salvage cryosurgery for recurrent prostate cancer after radiation therapy: a seven-year follow-up. *Clin Prostate Cancer* 2003;2: 111–114.

8. Ng CK, et al. Salvage cryoablation of the prostate: followup and analysis of predictive factors for outcome. *J Urol* 2007;178: 1253–1257; discussion 1257.

9. Ismail M, et al. Salvage cryotherapy for recurrent prostate cancer after radiation failure: a prospective case series of the first 100 patients. *BJU Int* 2007;100: 760–764.

10. Pisters LL, et al. Salvage prostate cryoablation: initial results from the cryo on-line data registry. *J Urol* 2008;180: 559–563.

11. Gowardhan B, Greene D. Salvage cryotherapy: is there a role for focal therapy? J *Endourol* 2010; 24(5): 861–864.

12. Eisenberg ML, Shinohara K. Partial salvage cryoablation of the prostate for recurrent prostate cancer after radiotherapy failure. *Urology* 2008;72: 1315–1318.

13. Spiess PE, et al. Presalvage prostate-specific antigen (PSA) and PSA doubling time as predictors of biochemical failure of salvage cryotherapy in patients with locally recurrent prostate cancer after radiotherapy. *Cancer* 2006;107: 275–280.

14. Gheiler EL, et al. Predictors for maximal outcome in patients undergoing salvage surgery for radio-recurrent prostate cancer. *Urology* 1998;51: 789–795.

15. Huang WC, et al. The anatomical and pathological characteristics of irradiated prostate cancers may influence the oncological efficacy of salvage ablative therapies. *J Urol* 2007;177(4): 1324–1329.

16. Cellini N, et al. Analysis of intraprostatic failures in patients treated with hormonal therapy and radiotherapy: Implications for conformal therapy planning. *IJROBP* 2002;53: 595–599.

17. Arumainayagam N, et al. Accuracy of multiparametric magnetic resonance imaging in detecting recurrent prostate cancer after radiotherapy. *BJUInt* 2010;106(7): 991–997.

18. Sartor AO, et al. Evaluating localized prostate cancer and identifying candidates for focal therapy. *Urology* 2008;72: S12–S24.

CHAPTER 12

High-Intensity Focused Ultrasound

Hashim U. Ahmed MRCS BM BCh BA(Hons)[1], and Mark Emberton FRCS (Urol)FRCS MD MBBS BSc[1,2]

[1]Division of Surgery and Interventional Science, University College London, London, UK
[2]NIHR UCL/UCH Comprehensive Biomedical Research Centre, London, UK

Introduction

Ultrasound refers to mechanical vibrations above the threshold of human hearing (16 kHz), which has the ability to interact with tissue to produce biological changes. The sound waves are generated by applying an alternating voltage across a piezoelectric material such as lead zirconate titanate: these materials oscillate at the same frequency as the alternating current causing ultrasound wave that can propagate through tissues. This in turn causes alternating cycles of increased and reduced pressure (compression and rarefaction, respectively). Diagnostic ultrasound usually uses frequencies in the range of 1–20 MHz, but therapeutic ultrasound uses frequencies of 0.8–3.5 MHz with energy delivery within the ultrasound beams that are several times greater than the energy levels of diagnostic ultrasound. Therapeutic ultrasound can be conveniently divided into two broad categories: "low" intensity (0.125–3 W/cm^2) and "high" intensity (>5 W/cm^2). The former can stimulate normal physiological responses to injury and accelerate other processes such as the transport of drugs across the skin. High-intensity ultrasound can selectively destroy tissue if delivered in a focused manner (high-intensity focused ultrasound (HIFU)) [1].

HIFU relies on the physical properties of ultrasound, which allow it to be brought into a tight focus either using an acoustic lens, bowl-shaped transducer, or electronic-phased array. As ultrasound propagates through a tissue so that zones of high- and low-pressure are created. When the energy density at the focus is sufficiently high (during the high-pressure phase), tissue damage occurs. The volume of ablation (or lesion) following a single HIFU pulse or exposure is small and varies according to transducer characteristics. It is typically shaped like a grain of rice or cigar with dimensions in the order of 1–3 mm (transverse) by 8–15 mm (along beam axis). To ablate larger volumes of tissue for the treatment of solid cancers, these lesions are placed adjacent to each other with a degree of overlap. The two predominant mechanisms of tissue damage are by the conversion of mechanical energy into heat and "inertial cavitation." If tissue temperatures are raised above 56°C, then immediate thermal toxicity can occur, provided the temperature is maintained for at least 1 second. This will lead to irreversible cell death from coagulative necrosis. In fact, during HIFU the temperatures achieved are much greater than this, typically above 80°C, so even short exposures can lead to effective cell death. Inertial cavitation occurs at the same time but is neither as controllable nor predictable. It occurs due to the alternating cycles of compression and rarefaction. At the time of rarefaction, gas can be drawn out of solution to form bubbles, which then collapse rapidly. The mechanical stress and a degree of thermal injury induce cell necrosis [2].

Histologically, the tissue changes that occur are homogeneous coagulative necrosis, with an inflammatory response that follows leading to formation of granulation tissue—indicated by the presence of immature fibroblasts and new capillary formation—at the periphery of the necrotic area at about a week after treatment. Polymorphonuclear leukocytes migrate deep into the treated tissue and then at 2 weeks, the boundary of the treated region is replaced by proliferative repair tissue.

The placement of the small HIFU lesions requires precise planning for an entire tumor to be ablated reliably. Furthermore, patient movement can lead to areas of viable malignant tissue remaining after treatment and even in ideal situations other factors can prevent a successful treatment. The most important of these include the heat-sink effect and calcification. The heat-sink effect relates to one area that overheats in the HIFU-pulse pathway and thus prevents adequate ultrasound propagation to the targeted area—such a phenomenon occurs if the time between HIFU pulses is inadequate for tissue cooling or if an area is high in water content, such as a cyst. In addition, highly vascularized tissues might be more resistant to thermal ablation owing to the heat-sink effect of their blood supply. Calcification simply leads to reverberation and shielding of the targeted area from parts of the HIFU pulse leading to inadequate heating of the tissue.

HIFU devices

Currently, there are two commercially available transrectal devices that can treat the prostate gland, the Ablatherm® device (Edap-Technomed, Lyon, France) and the Sonablate® 500 (Focus Surgery, Indianapolis, IN,

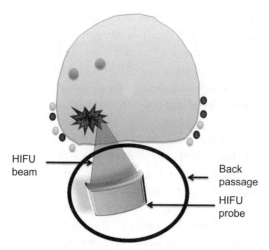

HIFU
beam

Back
passage

HIFU
probe

Figure 12.1 Transrectal HIFU devices can ablate prostate tissue with the beam
traversing the rectum and causing minimal harm to the intervening structures.

USA) (Figure 12.1). Ultrasound guidance, built-in safety features, and de-
gassed chilled water (17–20°C) are pumped through the system in order
to prevent rectal wall injury by heat build-up. A transurethral HIFU device has been designed and is undergoing phase I preclinical animal studies with planned early phase I human studies at the time of writing. A
MRI-guided device is also undergoing early phase I studies. Therefore, this
chapter will be limited to the two widely available devices.

The Ablatherm® until very recently had separate imaging (7 MHz) and
therapy transducers (3 MHz), which had a fixed focal length of 4 cm.
Prostate imaging during treatment was not possible but performed between treatment zones by inserting the imaging transducer through the
therapeutic transducer. The latest modification to the Ablatherm combines
treatment and planning probes so that visual feedback is possible during
treatment. However, because the Ablatherm uses algorithm-driven treatment protocols with preset energy levels, individual pulse energy levels
cannot be modified by the operator. Other features include the incorpora-
tion of the probe into a table that holds the pump and cooling mechanism
and upon which the patient is placed in the right lateral position. Treatment is to each lobe in turn and performed anterior to posterior within a
complete block that incorporates the full anterior-posterior height of the
prostate. A number of safety features that monitor the rectal wall energy
deposition are in place to prevent damage to this area. Many centers that
use Ablatherm combine transurethral resection of the prostate or bladder
neck incision in order to reduce gland size and stricture formation. It is
likely that the Ablatherm can carry out hemiablation or zonal ablation but
not focal ablation.

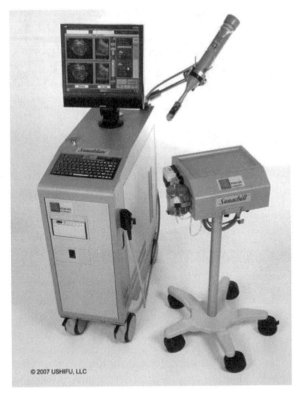

© 2007 USHIFU, LLC

Figure 12.2 The Sonablate 500 transrectal HIFU probe and transducer. (Courtesy of UKHIFU Ltd, UK.)

The Sonablate® system consists of a rectal probe (containing the transducer) with an operating frequency of 4 MHz that attempts to optimize the combined imaging and therapy roles of the transducer (Figure 12.2). This has the advantage of allowing visualization of treatment effect following each pulse of the treatment cycle. Rectal wall monitoring features are also in place with this probe. Treatment planning, execution, and monitoring are controlled using a user interface that allows the surgeon to precisely target the area of treatment, adjust the focal length of the transducer (currently 3 cm, 4 cm, or 4.5 cm), and alter the power intensity delivered to each focal zone individually. Rather than a protocol driven treatment, the power intensity of each pulse is guided by gray scale changes within the targeted area that represent steam, so that greater certainty about cell kill is obtained (Figure 12.3). The Sonablate 500 delivers treatment to the prostate in three separate blocks. The anterior portion of the prostate is treated initially, followed by midzone, and then posterior gland. Errors can arise as the probe requires adjustment between each of these blocks. The posterior block is always treated using the 3-cm focal length and with

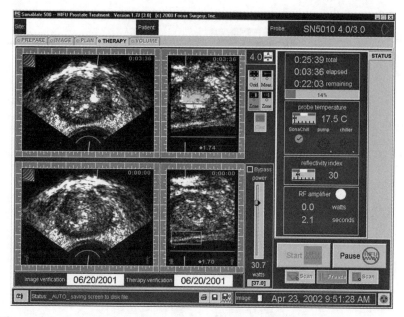

Figure 12.3 Screen capture demonstrating what the operator sees during a Sonablate 500 treatment. (Courtesy of UKHIFU Ltd, UK.) (See Plate 12.3.)

lower energy levels. Within each zone, multiple overlapping lesions are created to enhance ablation (Figure 12.4). This device will allow hemiablation, zonal ablation, and focal ablation.

Focal therapy series

A number of studies are now emerging reporting on the safety, feasibility, toxicity, and early cancer control of focal therapy using HIFU

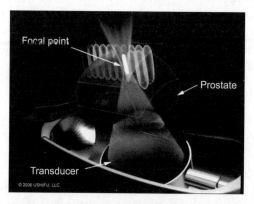

Figure 12.4 Diagrammatic representation of HIFU pulses delivered. Rows of pulses adjacent to each other are used to ablate larger areas of prostate. (Courtesy of UKHIFU Ltd, UK.) (See Plate 12.4.)

Table 12.1 Studies evaluating focal therapy of prostate cancer using HIFU.

	Muto et al. [3]	El Fegoun [4]	Ahmed et al. [5]	Ahmed et al. [5]
No.	29	12	20	43
Type of study	Retrospective	Retrospective	Prospective phase I/II trial	Prospective phase I/II trial
Device	Sonablate 500	Ablatherm	Sonablate 500	Sonablate 500
Localization	TRUS biopsy	TRUS biopsy	Multiparametric MRI and template mapping	Multiparametric MRI and template Mapping
Therapy	Hemiablation	Hemiablation	Hemiablation	Focal/zonal ablation
PSA (ng/mL), mean (range)	5 (range 2–25)	<10	7.3 (4.4–11.8)	7.4 (3.6–15.2)
Gleason score	≤8	≤7	≤7	≤7
Potency, %	Not reported	Not reported	95	80–100
Continence (pad-free), %	Not reported	100	95	100
Continence (leak-free, pad-free)	Not reported	Not reported	90	100
Disease control	76.5% (no cancer) (biopsy) (12 months)	58% (10 years)	90% (no cancer) 100% (no significant cancer) (Biopsy) (12 months)	79% (no cancer) 90% (no significant cancer) (Biopsy) (12 months)

(Table 12.1). The first series to report on focal HIFU was from Japan. Muto et al. (2008) reported on hemiablation using the Sonablate 500 HIFU device in a small retrospective case series that was mixed with whole-gland treated patients [3]. Twenty-nine patients who were found to have uni lateral disease on the basis of TRUS biopsy were treated to ablation of both peripheral zones and one half of the transition zone. Ten percent (3/28) had positive biopsies at 6 months, whereas 23.5% (4/17) had further positive biopsies at 12 months. There was no significant change in the IPSS score for urinary symptoms, although there was one urethral stricture and one urinary tract infection. Although demonstrating feasibility of focal therapy using a transrectal HIFU device, the reporting in this series was very poor and the group tried to make comparison to a nonrandomized group that were treated with whole-gland HIFU. Furthermore, they made no comment on the erectile function rate. Barret et al. (2008) reported their series of 12 men treated over a period of about 10–15 years.

This retrospective series has only been published in abstract form and is therefore incomplete in its data and poorly reported.

A number of prospective clinical trials are now reporting. Ahmed et al. have shown that hemiablation using the Sonablate 500 in 20 men characterized by multiparametric MRI and template prostate mapping carried an early return of baseline genitourinary function by 3–6 months with 95% having erections sufficient for intercourse (one-third requiring phosphodiesterase inhibitors), 95% being pad-free, and 90% being pad-free and leak-free. Biopsy of the treated areas showed no cancer in 90% and no significant cancer (<1 core positive, Gleason 3+3, ≤3 mm) in all men biopsied [5]. PSA levels decreased by about 80% by 3–6 months. Another study by Ahmed et al. showed that HIFU focal/zonal ablation in 42 bilateral low- to intermediate-risk men with cancer (using the exact same trial design as the earlier study) could achieve encouraging genitourinary functional return and early cancer control [6]. The slightly lower figures in this trial may be related to the increased precision required in focal ablation not achieving the margin of treatment that hemiablation can achieve. Further trials by this group are ongoing. The Lesion Control HIFU study aims to ablate only the index (largest by volume and highest grade) lesion in 56 men using HIFU and the INDEX trial is an international multicenter study of 135 men in which all the above trial protocols are incorporated, but in addition template mapping biopsies are repeated at 3 years to determine whether untreated lesions progress in the medium term.

Conclusion

HIFU may have the necessary attributes required for the focal treatment of prostate cancer. It is minimally invasive, and certainly requires from puncture of epithelial surfaces, is precise, controllable, repeatable, and can be carried out in an ambulatory day-case setting. Early trials are demonstrated very encouraging outcomes for function and side effects but cancer control will need to be assessed in medium- to long-term studies to determine whether it has a place in standard care.

References

1. Hill CR, ter Haar GR. Review article: high intensity focused ultrasound–potential for cancer treatment. *Br J Radiol* 1995;68(816): 1296–1303.
2. Kennedy JE. High-intensity focused ultrasound in the treatment of solid tumours. *Nat Rev Cancer* 2005;5(4): 321–327.
3. Muto S et al. Focal therapy with high-intensity-focused ultrasound in the treatment of localized prostate cancer. *Jpn J Clin Oncol* 2008;38(3): 192–199.

4. El Fegoun et al. Int Braz *J Urol* 2011;37(2): 213–222.

5. Ahmed HU et al. Focal Therapy for Localized Prostate Cancer: A Phase I/II Trial. *J Urol* 2011;185(4): 1246–1254.

6. Ahmed HU et al. Focal therapy of prostate cancer using high intensity focused ultrasound (Sonablate500TM)—interim results from two Phase II trials. *2nd International Workshop on Imaging and Focal Therapy of Renal and Prostate Cancer;* 2010, Washington.

CHAPTER 13

Energies for Focal Ablation: Photodynamic Therapy

Caroline M. Moore MD MRCS(Ed)[1], Nimalan Arumainayagam MD[2], and Mark Emberton FRCS (Urol) FRCS MD MBBS BSc[2,3]

[1]University College London and University College London Hopsitals NHS Trust, London, UK
[2]Division of Surgery and Interventional Sciences, University College London, London, UK
[3]NIHR UCL/UCH Comprehensive Biomedical Research Centre, London, UK

Introduction

Photodynamic therapy (PDT) uses a photosensitizing drug, activated by light, in the presence of oxygen to ablate tissue. In 1978, Dougherty published a clinical series of the use of PDT for a range of subcutaneous or metastatic cancers [1], declaring "no type to be unresponsive." In 1990, the first clinical report of PDT for localized prostate cancer was seen [2]. Other groups then began to investigate the use of different photosensitizers, in preclinical and clinical studies.

Mechanism of action

PDT uses a photosensitizing drug, given in an inactive state, and activated after a period of time—the drug light interval—by light of a specific wavelength, in the presence of oxygen. Each of the three components, drug, light, and oxygen, must be present for the photodynamic effect to occur. The drug can be given topically—for skin conditions, such as acne or skin cancers—orally or intravenously. Photosensitizers differ in their drug light interval, wavelength of activation, and photodynamic efficiency, i.e., the effect produced for a given concentration of drug.

The photosensitizer is administered in a stable form (ground state). It is then promoted to a higher energy state (singlet state) by light of a specific wavelength (Figure 13.1). The excited photosensitizer is then unstable and can release energy in one of the three ways: emission of heat or light, or

---

Focal Therapy in Prostate Cancer, First Edition. Edited by Hashim U Ahmed, Manit Arya, Peter Carroll and Mark Emberton.

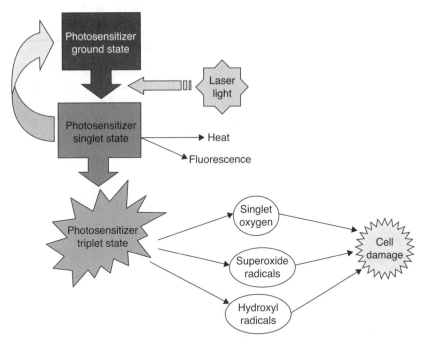

Figure 13.1   Schematic showing mechanism of action of photodynamic therapy. The photosensitizer is administered in a stable form (ground state) and promoted to a higher energy state (singlet state) by light of a specific wavelength. The excited photosensitizer is then unstable and can release energy in one of three ways: emission of heat or light, or conversion to an intermediate energy state (triplet state), before returning to stable ground state. In triplet state, the photosensitizer can produce hydroxyl and superoxide radicals (type 1 reaction), or convert molecular tissue oxygen to form singlet oxygen (type 2 reaction). This singlet oxygen in turn reacts with proteins, lipids, and nucleic acids in cells, causing functional and structural damage, which leads to cell death. Hydroxyl and superoxide radicals are also directly responsible for cell death.

conversion to an intermediate energy state (triplet state), before returning to stable ground state. In triplet state, the photosensitizer can produce hydroxyl and superoxide radicals (type 1 reaction), or convert molecular tissue oxygen to form singlet oxygen (type 2 reaction). This singlet oxygen in turn reacts with proteins, lipids, and nucleic acids in cells causing functional and structural damage, which leads to cell death. Hydroxyl and superoxide radicals are also directly responsible for cell death. It is likely that the immune response to PDT is also important in its effect, although this requires further clinical study.

Tissue activated photosensitizers are activated when they have reached sufficient concentration in the target tissue, with some accumulating preferentially in tumor tissue; this can take several hours or days. These photosensitizers tend to accumulate in the skin and eyes, where activation by ambient light can cause a sunburn-like reaction.

Vascular-activated photosensitizers can be activated within a few min-utes of intravenous administration, and, due to rapid clearance, tend not to be found in the skin or eyes for more than a couple of hours. The differ-ent photosensitizers that have been used in clinical and preclinical prostate work are summarized in Table 13.1. The ideal photosensitizer would have a short drug light interval, allowing treatment in a single clinical session; a long activation wavelength allowing deep penetration into tissue; a pre-dictable effect for a given drug and light dose; and no accumulation in the skin [3].

Technique of prostate photodynamic therapy

Depending on the drug light interval, the photosensitizer can either be given prior to hospital attendance for the light administration or in the same clinical session. Light is usually produced by a laser, commonly a diode laser, and delivered using optical delivery fibers. These can either be bare-ended fibers (so that light is emitted from the end, like a torch), or cylindrically diffusing fibers (which emit light at the distal 1–4 cm, like a strip-light) (Figure 13.2). The laser fibers are placed within the prostate, usually within blind-ended hollow plastic needles. The needles are placed using transrectal ultrasound and a perineal template, in a similar manner to brachytherapy delivery (Figure 13.3).

The procedure is performed under general anesthetic in the lithotomy position. Typically, a urinary catheter is placed during the procedure and removed the next day. Protecting the skin and eyes from light during the procedure is necessary, and is continued after drug administration, and until the drug is cleared (up to 6 weeks for tissue-based photosensitiz-ers such as mTHPC; a few hours for vascular-activated photosensitizers). Monitoring of light levels in the prostate, urethra, and rectum can help in modifying the light dose to avoid unwanted extraprostatic effects.

Preclinical studies

A number of groups have studied different photosensitizers in benign ca-nine prostates. When using tin ethyl etiopurin (SnET2), delivering light ei-ther by the transperineal or transurethral route, it was shown that higher photosensitizer concentrations were seen in the prostate compared to rectum, urethra and bladder. PDT studies showed hemorrhagic necrosis around the light fibers, with a mean radius of 6 mm. Serial studies showed that although urethral mucosa was initially absent following treatment, by 6 weeks complete urethral regeneration had occurred. Rectal damage

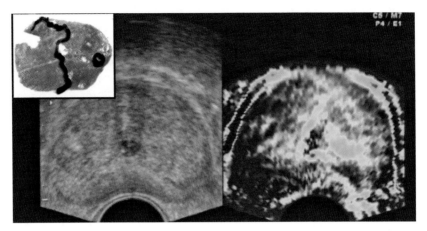

Plate 6.1 Ultrasound real-time elastography or strain imaging. Prostate cancer can hardly be detected using the conventional B-mode image alone. The strain image or elastogram on the right depicts stiff areas in red to black. Soft areas are colored yellow to blue. (See Fig. 6.1.)

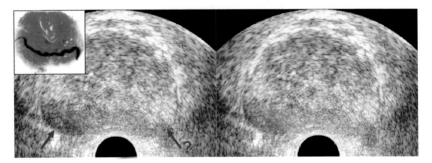

Plate 6.2 Ultrasound tissue characterization. Areas of the prostate exhibiting high cancer probability are marked in red. Not only the right part of the tumor (arrow) was highlighted by the classification system but nearly the whole extension of the cancerous region was also detected. (See Fig. 6.2.)

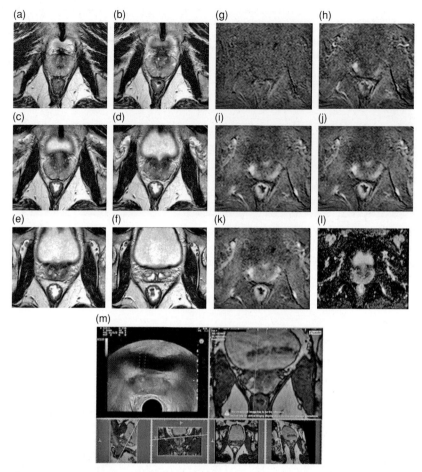

Plate 7.2 Patient with a history of slowly increasing PSA levels (currently 6.5 ng/mL) and two negative 12-core biopsies performed five (PSA 3.7 ng/mL in 2005) and 4 years earlier (PSA 4.4 ng/mL in 2006). DRE results were normal. A T2W MRI scan (images (a–f)) showed a small, 30-cc prostate, with diffuse homogeneous low signal intensity, but no suspicious lesion. A subtracted DCE-MRI scan performed on a 1.5T device equipped with an HRPPA coil revealed a significant 13 × 10 mm suspicious area in the right lateral base (images (g–k)) were taken in the same plane as image (d); (g) is unenhanced, (h) is the earliest enhanced image, and images (i–k) are subsequent enhanced images acquired every 15 seconds). A diffusion-weighted scan in the same plane as the lesion (image (l)) did not reveal any anomaly. All systematic posterior biopsies (12 cores) were negative, but both additional DCE-MRI-guided targeted biopsies under image fusion (m) were positive for adenocarcinoma (Gleason 3 + 4 = 7). (See Fig. 7.2.)

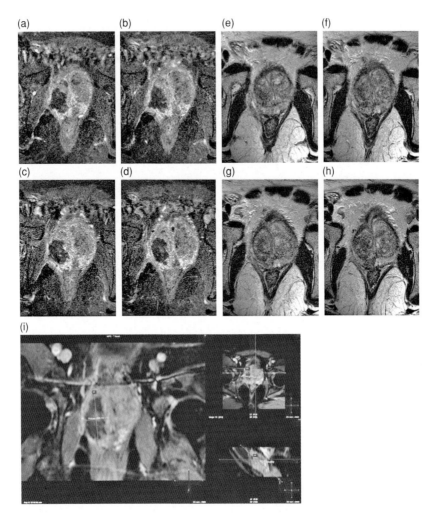

Plate 7.3 DCE-MRI performed 7 days after vascular-targeted photodynamic therapy (VTP). The patient had an initial PSA of 8.3 ng/mL, with only one positive core out of 12 (Gleason 3 + 3 = 6) at biopsy, in the right median lobe. Images (a–d) show four consecutive slices of the treated gland in a late (4 minutes postinjection) three-dimensional DCE-MRI scan performed on a 1.5T device using an HRPPA coil and fat saturation. They clearly show a well-circumscribed hypovascularized area corresponding to the treated zone (right posterior lobe). Images (e–h) are corresponding T2W slices, showing only large areas of low intensity, with unclear margins. Image (i) illustrates the advantage of using multiplanar reconstruction to assess treated areas. (See Fig. 7.3.)

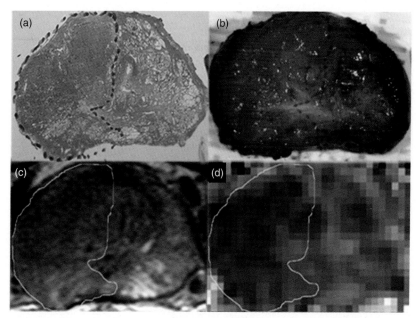

Plate 8.2 (a) Hematoxylin and eosin-stained histology section from a whole-mount prostatectomy specimen (b) showing tumor outline (in blue). On the T2W image in (c), this tumor outline (in yellow) has been warped to fit the T2W image slice and then overlaid onto the ADC map in (d). The tumor has lower ADC compared to the normal left peripheral zone. (See Fig. 8.2.) (Reprinted with permission from Extra-Cranial Applications of Diffusion-Weighted MRI, Edited by Bachir Taouli, 2010, © Cambridge University Press)

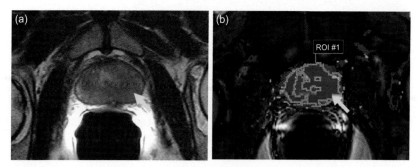

Plate 9.1 Dynamic contrast-enhanced MRI detection of prostate cancer. T2-weighted (a) and DCE MRI K_{trans} maps (b) demonstrate a tumor in the left-peripheral zone that was proven to be prostate cancer by histology. The elevation in K_{trans} exhibited by the tumor is thought to reflect increased vascular permeability and surface area associated with tumor neovascularization. (See Fig. 9.1.)

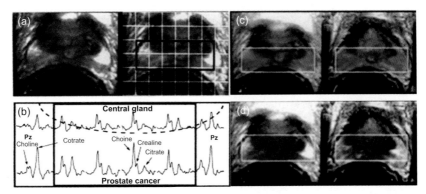

Plate 9.2 MR spectroscopy of prostate cancer. MRI and MR spectroscopy performed on a 48 year old male with an elevated PSA demonstrate a T2 hypointense mass (a; circle) occupying the peripheral zone of the left mid gland with an irregular prostate capsule. Multivoxel MR spectroscopy (b) demonstrates an elevated choline:citrate in multiple voxels (circle) corresponding to the mass. A Gleason grade 9 adenocarcinoma at this location was found at surgery. Images courtesy of Sadhna Verma, MD. (See Fig. 9.2.)

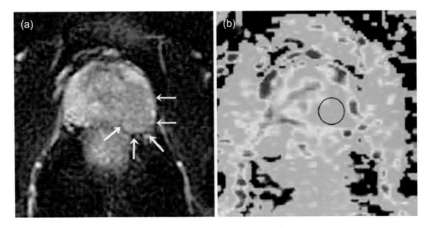

Plate 9.3 MR diffusion-weighted imaging of prostate cancer. T2-weighted (a) and apparent diffusion coefficient (ADC) maps (b) from a 58-year-old male with known prostate cancer demonstrate restricted diffusion (circle) corresponding to the region of the patient's biopsy-proved left-peripheral zone tumor (arrows). (From Tamada T, et al. Apparent diffusion coefficient values in peripheral and transition zones of the prostate: comparison between normal and malignant prostatic tissues and correlation with histologic grade. *JMRI* 2008; **28:**720–726, reproduced with permission of John Wiley & Sons, Inc.) (See Fig. 9.3.)

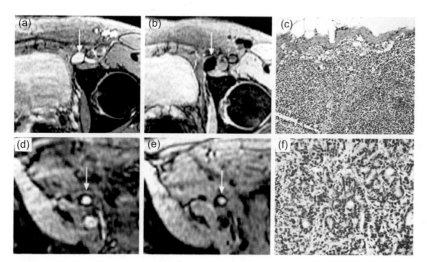

Plate 9.4 LN-MRI detection of prostate cancer metastasis. T2-weighted MRI images of lymph nodes in prostate cancer patients are shown before (a, d) and after (b, e) administration of USPIO, as well as representative histology (c, f) from the lymph nodes after surgical resection. The top row shows a benign lymph node (c) that demonstrates signal loss following USPIO administration (b). The bottom row shows a malignant lymph node (f) that does not accumulate USPIO (e). (From Harisinghani MG, et al. Noninvasive detection of clinically occult lymph-node metastases in prostate cancer. *NEJM* 2003; 348:2491–2499, reproduced with permission. Copyright © 2003 Massachusetts Medical Society, all rights reserved.) (See Fig. 9.4.)

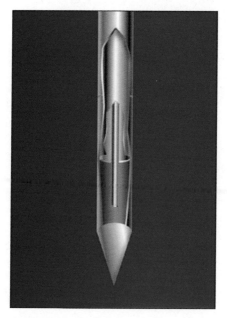

Plate 10.1 Engineering drawing of gas-driven cryoprobe. Use of gas rather than liquid allowed for smaller needle diameter and subsequently direct prostate access. The Joule–Thomson effect allows the single cryoprobe to both cool and warm the tissue by using Argon and Helium gasses, respectively. (See Fig. 10.1.)

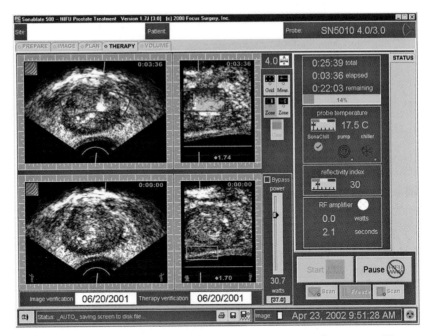

Plate 12.3 Screen capture demonstrating what the operator sees during a Sonablate 500 treatment. (Courtesy of UKHIFU Ltd, UK.) (See Fig. 12.3.)

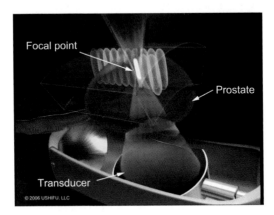

Plate 12.4 Diagrammatic representation of HIFU pulses delivered. Rows of pulses adjacent to each other are used to ablate larger areas of prostate. (Courtesy of UKHIFU Ltd, UK.) (See Fig. 12.4.)

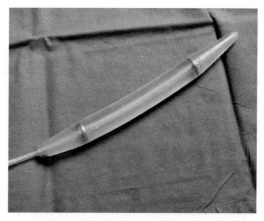

Plate 13.2 Photograph of a cylindrical diffuser. A cylindrically diffusing optical fiber, which emits light along a defined distance, usually between 1 cm and 4 cm. (See Fig. 13.2.)

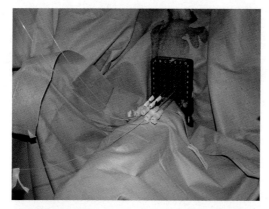

Plate 13.3 Prostate PDT procedure. With the patient in lithotomy position, the perineal template can be clearly seen. The ultrasound probe is covered by the sterile drape. The hollow plastic needles are within the prostate, and the optical fibers inserted within the needles, and attached to the laser and optical detector. (See Fig. 13.3.)

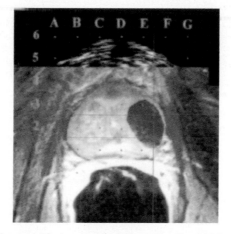

Plate 14.1 MRI-ultrasound fusion used for biopsy. (See Fig. 14.1.)

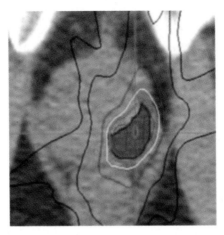

Plate 14.2 Dose distribution using CyberKnife to focally boost radiation dose using MRI to define dominant lesion. (See Fig. 14.2.)

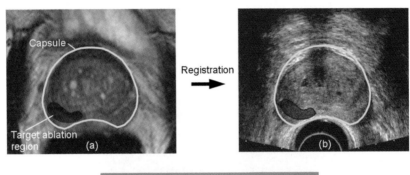

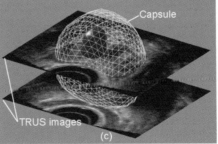

Plate 15.1 (a) A slice through a T2-weighted MR volume of the prostate with a target region for focal ablation shown in red. (b) Registered TRUS image with the MR-derived therapy plan overlaid. (c) Three-dimensional representation of an MR-derived therapy plan registered with a TRUS image volume (only two slices of this volume are shown for clarity). Once registered, the therapy plan can be used in conjunction with intraoperative TRUS images to aid precise therapy delivery. (See Fig. 15.1.)

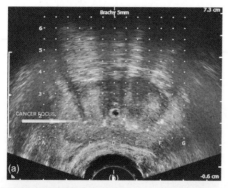

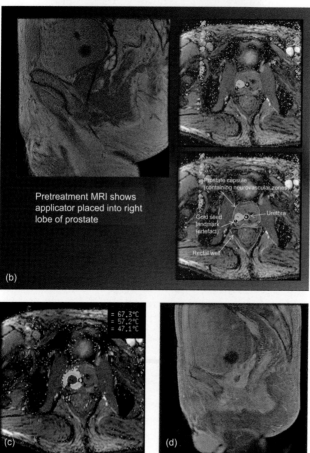

Plate 16.1 Series of figures demonstrating a focal therapy using an interstitial photothermal ablative therapy with an in-bore MRI. Template-mapping biopsies located the cancer in the right lobe of the prostate (a); the applicator was placed accurately into this area during treatment and verified on MRI (b); real-time feedback using MRI thermometry is possible to ensure adequate ablation limited to the targeted area (c); early verification using a postgadolinium contrast MRI demonstrating perfusion deficit in the treated area (d). (See Fig. 16.1.)

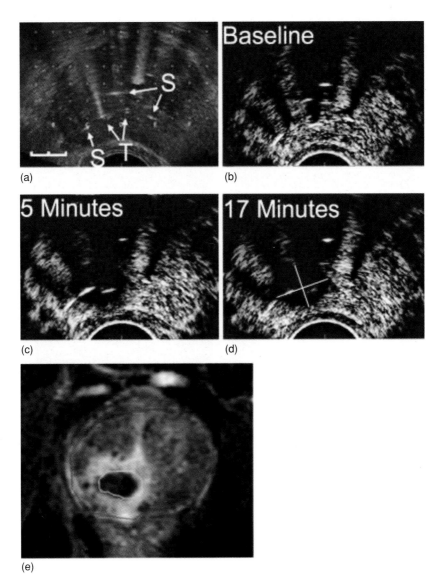

Plate 17.1 Evolving perfusion defect on contrast-enhanced ultrasound during interstitial laser thermotherapy. (a) A transverse ultrasound image for treatment planning. T marks treatment fibers and S sensory fibers. (b–d) Contrast-enhanced (0.2 mL Definity, Lantheus Medical Imaging, N. Billerica, MA, USA) ultrasound images before and 5 and 17 minutes after the start of treatment. (e) The corresponding contrast-enhanced MRI showing an equivalent defect in enhancement 7 days after treatment. The circle corresponds to the defect seen on ultrasound. (By kind permission of Drs R Weersink, M Gertner, and J Trachtenberg and the *Canadian Urological Association Journal*.) (See Fig. 17.1.)

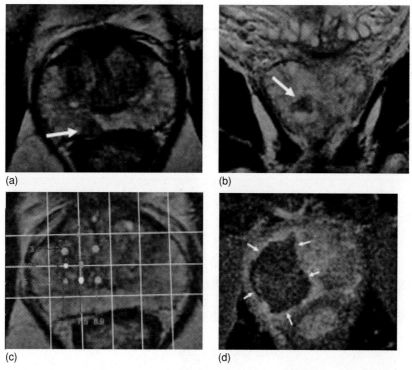

Plate 17.4 Planning and early appearances after focal photodynamic therapy. (a, b) Axial and coronal T2-weighted images, respectively, showing the tumor (white arrow). (c) The treatment planning image, with positions for fiber placement. (d) A postcontrast T1-weighted axial image showing the resulting area of confluent necrosis at 7 days (white arrows). (See Fig. 17.4.)

Table 13.1 Comparison of different photosensitizers used clinically.

Photosensitizer	Optimum dose	Route of administration	Drug light interval	Activating wavelength	Comments
Hematoporphyrin-derivative (HpD)	1.5 mg/kg	Intravenous	Days	630 nm	One of first photosensitizers in clinical use difficult to manufacture reliably; prolonged skin sensitivity
Porfirmer derivative (Photofrin)	2.5 mg/kg	Intravenous	Days	630 nm	Commercial preparation of HpD—less heterogeneous; prolonged skin sensitivity.
Meso tetra hydroxy phenyl chlorin (mTHPC, Foscan)	0.15 mg/kg	Intravenous	3–5 days	652 nm	High quantum yield, i.e., low drug dose required to produce photodynamic effect; prolonged skin sensitivity
Motexafin lutetium (MLu, LuTex)	2 mg/kg	Intravenous	3 hours	730 or 732 nm	Shorter drug light interval (3 hours); no reported skin sensitivity
ALA (amino levulinic acid)	20 mg/kg	Oral	3–6 hours	635 nm	Selectivity for cancer in radical prostatectomy study
WST-09 (Tookad, palladium bactereopheophorobide, not water soluble)	2 mg/kg	Intravenous	10 minutes	763 nm	Short drug light interval (minutes); no skin photosensitivity after 3 hours; effectiveness proven with PSA and imaging.
WST-11 (Palladium bactereopheophorbide, water soluble)	4–6 mg/kg	Intravenous	10 minutes	753 nm	Does not require Cremaphor for administration; predictable PDT effect

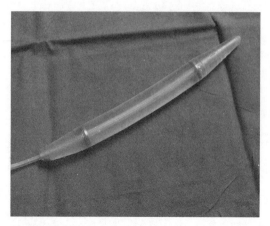

Figure 13.2 Photograph of a cylindrical diffuser. A cylindrically diffusing optical fiber, which emits light along a defined distance, usually between 1 cm and 4 cm. (See Plate 13.2.)

was seen in two animals, where the light diffuser was within 5 mm of the rectum. The necrotic lesions appeared to resolve with atrophy and fibrosis, leading to prostate volume reduction. Minimal side effects were noted, with all animals voiding spontaneously.

This group, while never translating their results to clinical studies, did do some complex modeling of photosensitizer distribution, light penetration, and PDT effect, and were able to predict necrosis in the canine model to within 2 mm. It would have been very interesting to see if the same technique could have been used clinically. Other photosensitizers used in

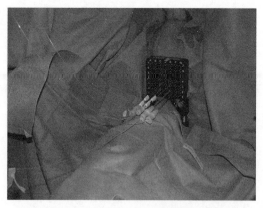

Figure 13.3 Prostate PDT procedure. With the patient in lithotomy position, the perineal template can be clearly seen. The ultrasound probe is covered by the sterile drape. The hollow plastic needles are within the prostate, and the optical fibers inserted within the needles, and attached to the laser and optical detector. (See Plate 13.3.)

the benign canine model were 5-aminolevulinic acid (ALA), motexafin lutetium, aluminium phthalocyanine (AlS2Pc), porfimer sodium, meso-tetra hydroxyphenyl chlorin (mTHPC), and palladium bacteriopheophorbide (WST-09).

The group using WST-09 in the normal canine prostate also assessed its use following radiation therapy, and in spontaneous prostate cancer in the dog. They concluded that it was safe and effective even following radiotherapy in this model. They also compared the effect seen on 1 week MRI with whole-mount radical prostatectomy, and noted good correlation between treatment volumes [4]. They also assessed the effect of WST-09 PDT on nerves, showing that peripheral nerves were relatively resistant to PDT at doses that caused ablation elsewhere. Preclinical work established the most effective drug and light doses for a number of different photosensitizers, which were then used in clinical studies.

Clinical studies of PDT for prostate cancer

Studies in radiorecurrent prostate cancer

The first formal clinical study of PDT for prostate cancer was reported by the groups at University College London, who had explored a number of photosensitizers in the canine model. They used mTHPC in men with recurrent prostate cancer following radiotherapy [5]. Five men were treated at a low light dose, with no apparent effect, and 13 men (including four of the original five) at a higher light dose. Drug light intervals of 3–5 days and a combination of bare-ended fibers and cylindrical diffusers were used. Patchy effects were seen on posttreatment cross-sectional imaging, and were associated with a reduction in PSA and negative biopsies in some men. PSA began to rise in all men, and androgen therapy was started at a mean of 10 months after PDT. Most men had some irritative urinary symptoms in the first month, and of the seven men who had some sexual function prior to PDT, only three maintained this afterward. One man had a rectal biopsy of abnormal mucosa 1 month after PDT, which led to the formation of a urethrorectal fistula, requiring a temporary colostomy. Five men had mild skin sensitivity reactions, which resolved spontaneously.

Motexafin lutetium has also been used in radiorecurrent prostate cancer, using a range of drug doses, drug light intervals, and light doses. It was found that the higher drug dose of 2 mg/kg, activated by 200 J/cm², resulted in the greatest initial rise in PSA, and the greatest delay to biochemical progression. There was a variability of response in this small patient group, which could be overcome by individualized treatment planning on the basis of photosensitizer concentrations in the prostate, and measurement of optical properties (absorption and scattering of light in the prostate) prior to light delivery. As these studies did not report any MRI findings following PDT, which would have been useful in assessing the extent of the PDT effect, it is likely that there was only moderate ablation.

Trachtenberg and colleagues reported their work in radiorecurrent prostate cancer using the vascular-activated photosensitizer, WST-09 [6]. They noted a threshold effect, where a light dose of 23 J/cm^2 in 90% of the volume resulted in a 60% complete response, i.e., 60% of the men had extensive avascular lesions on 1 week MRI and a biopsy negative for cancer at 6 months. There was only transient urinary toxicity and no skin sensitivity. Two of the men developed rectourethral fistula, with one of these resolving with catheterization, and the other causing intermittent problems at 6-month follow-up (Table 13.2).

Clinical work in primary prostate cancer

The first clinical report of PDT for primary prostate cancer reported two men who had PDT 6 weeks after two transurethral resections of the prostate. One received hematoporphyrins derivative, and the other porfimer sodium. The photosensitizer was given intravenously and activated using 638-nm laser light delivered with a spherical tip fiber. Random biopsy at 3 months showed no cancer and PSA was reduced.

Studies on the photosensitizer ALA with photosensitizer prior to radical prostatectomy showed a differential uptake of the drug in cancer as opposed to benign tissue. Further work assessed the use of transurethral and transperineal light delivery in 6 men; a planned radical prostatectomy in one man showed necrosis at the point of fiber insertion; in the other 5 men, PSA levels were seen to decrease, although post-PDT imaging was not carried out.

The University College London group used mTHPC in men as a first-line treatment [13]. This pilot study of 10 treatments in six men showed that the procedure was well tolerated, and resulted in a lowering of PSA associated with PDT effect seen on posttreatment MRI. However, this work was not developed as the drug manufacturer faced financial difficulties. This group is now investigating the use of palladium bactereopheophorbides in this patient population, within the setting of a European multicenter study (Table 13.3).

Use of PDT in focal treatment of prostate cancer

Treatment planning for prostate PDT, whether for focal or whole-gland treatment, is complex, requiring decisions about total drug dose, rate of

Table 13.2 Published clinical studies of PDT for radiorecurrent prostate cancer.

Reference	Photosensitizer (drug dose)	Light delivery: route dose wavelength	Drug–light interval	Target volume	Patient characteristics: Gleason score, PSA level Primary/salvage setting	Number of patients	Imaging results	Biopsy results	PSA response	Adverse effects	Limitations of the study
Nathan et al. [5]	Temoporfin (0.15 mg/kg iv)	Transperineal freehand insertion 20 or 50 J/cm² 652 nm	3 days	Less than whole gland	PSA before radiotherapy up to 37 ng/L	14	Up to 91% necrosis on CT	Negative biopsies in 3/14 patients	10/14 patients had a PSA level reduction by up to 96%	Rectourethral fistula after rectal biopsy Stress urinary incontinence Acute urinary retention	Freehand fiber placement Variable timing of posttreatment imaging Variable light dose
Pinthus et al. [7]; Verigos et al. [8]; Patel et al. [9]	Motexafin lutetium (0.50/1.00/ 2.00 mg/kg iv)	Perineal template 25–150 J/cm² 732 nm Computer-aided light-dose planning	3/6/24h	Whole gland	External beam (n = 8), Brachytherapy (n = 9)	17*	N/A	Negative biopsies in 3/14 patients	Transient rise then fall in high-dose PDT only PSA values were analyzed for only 14 of the 17 patients	1/14 grade II urinary urgency (catheter related) Grade I genitourinary symptoms in many	Posttreatment imaging and biopsy not reported Marked variation in PDT doses
Trachtenberg et al. [10]; Haider et al. [11]; Trachtenberg et al. [6]; Weersink et al. [12]	Padoporfin (0.10–2.00 mg/kg iv)	Perineal template, computer-aided light-dose planning Up to 360 J/cm 763 nm	10 min	Whole gland in multifiber patients; single fiber in each of the right and left lobes of the prostate in the earlier part of the study	Organ-confined recurrence after definitive radiotherapy	24 patients with light fibers; 28 patients with up to 6 fibers	Complete response on MRI in 60% of patients who received high drug and light dose	Complete response on biopsy in 60% of patients who received high drug and light dose	PSA levels decreased in the 8 patients who were biopsy-negative at 6 months	2 rectourethral fistulae 1 intraoperative hypotension Decreased urinary function until 6 months	Reason for heterogeneity in responses unclear

Table 13.3 Published clinical studies of PDT in primary prostate cancer.

Reference	Photosensitizer (drug dose)	Light delivery: route dose wavelength	Drug–light interval	Target volume	Patient characteristics: Gleason score PSA level Primary/salvage setting	Number of patients	Imaging results	Biopsy results	PSA response	Adverse effects	Limitations of the study
Windahl et al. [2]	Hematoporphyrin derivative (1.50 mg/kg iv)	Transurethral 15 J/cm² 638 nm	48 h	Post-TURP remnant	Post-TURP Primary setting	1	Posttreatment imaging not reported	Posttreatment biopsy not reported	Reduction in PSA level (10.0 to 2.5 µg/L)	No adverse effects reported	Posttreatment imaging and biopsy not reported Only one case reported
Windahl et al. [2]	Photofrin (2.50 mg/kg iv)	Transurethral 15 J/cm² 638 nm	72 h	Post-TURP remnant	Post-TURP Primary setting	1	Posttreatment imaging not reported	Posttreatment biopsy not reported	Reduction in PSA level (6.0 to 0.2 µg/L)	No adverse effects reported	Posttreatment imaging and biopsy not reported Only one case reported

Study	Drug (dose)	Time	Treatment area	Tumor characteristics	Necrosis/imaging	Histology	PSA response	Adverse effects
Moore et al. [7]	Temoporfin (0.15 mg/kg iv)	2–5 d	Less than whole gland	Gleason score 3+3 PSA level 1.9–15 ng/L 6 primary treatments 4 repeat treatments	Up to 51 cm^3 necrosis Residual cancer in all patients	Necrosis and fibrosis on biopsy	PSA reduction in 8/10 treatments	Gram negative sepsis ($n = 1$) irritative voiding symptoms for 2 wk 2 patients requiring re-catheterization Mild stress/urge incontinence ($n = 1$) Deterioration in erectile function ($n = 1$)
Zaak et al. [14]	Aminolevulinic acid-induced protoporphyrin IX (20.00 mg/kg orally)	4 h	1cm cylindrical diffuser Perineal ($n = 2$); transurethral ($n = 3$); radical prostatectomy $n = 1$) 250 J/cm 633 nm	Variable	Gleason score 5–8 PSA level 4.9–10.6 ng/mL Primary setting	Posttreatment imaging not reported	Necrosis observed on prostatectomy specimen at fiber insertion	Average decrease 55% for transurethral light delivery; 30% reduction for transperineal light delivery	No adverse effects reported

drug delivery, total light dose, light dose per cm of diffusing fiber, and rate of energy delivery. It is likely that there is a threshold effect, where sufficient light drug and oxygen must be present in a given volume of tissue, for necrosis to occur.

Treatment planning can be done with pretreatment MR and ultrasound volumes using a "rules-based" approach, where specific rules are set. For example, a 5 mm minimum distance from light delivery fiber to capsule, and a given energy density for a specific drug dose. Alternatively, it can be based on real-time feedback of drug, light, and oxygen measurements and the light dose modified accordingly throughout treatment. The first technique is being developed by those working with the palladium bactereophoeophorbide photosensitizers, while the second technique is being explored by the group in Lund [15]. Other possibilities are to attach a cancer-specific marker to a photosensitizer, which would then only be activated in areas of tumor. Although this concept has been explored in preclinical models, there has been no clinical work on such linked photosensitizers in prostate cancer to date.

While published studies to date have tended to use a variety of drug and light doses in a small number of men, larger studies are now being planned to assess the oncological efficacy of given drug and light doses in international multicenter studies [16]. The results of these will help to determine the place of PDT as one of the technologies used for focal treatment of prostate cancer in the coming years.

References

1. Dougherty TJ, et al. Photoradiation for the treatment of tumours. *Cancer Res* 1978;38: 2628–2635.
2. Windahl TF, et al. Photodynamic therapy of localised prostatic cancer. *Lancet* 1990;336(8723): 1139.
3. Moore CM, et al. Does photodynamic therapy have the necessary attributes to become a future treatment for organ-confined prostate cancer? *BJUInt* 2005;96(6): 754–758.
4. Huang Z, et al. Magnetic resonance imaging correlated with the histopathological effect of Pd-bacteriopheophorbide (Tookad) photodynamic therapy on the normal canine prostate gland. *Lasers Surg Med* 2006;38(7): 672–681.
5. Nathan TR, et al. Photodynamic therapy for prostate cancer recurrence after radiotherapy: a phase I study. J Urol 2002;168(4 Pt 1): 1427–1432.
6. Trachtenberg JF, et al. Vascular-targeted photodynamic therapy (padoporfin, WST09) for recurrent prostate cancer after failure of external beam radiotherapy: a study of escalating light doses. *BJUInt* 2008;102(5): 556–562.
7. Pinthus et al. *J Urol* 2006;175(4): 1201–1207.
8. Verigos et al. *J Environ Pathol Toxicol Oncol* 2006;25(1–2): 373–387.
9. Patel et al. *Clin Cancer Res* 2008;14(15): 4869–4876.

10. Trachtenberg et al. *BJU Int* 2004;94(2 Suppl): 57.

11. Haider et al. *Radiology* 2007;244(1): 196–204.

12.

13. Moore CM, et al. Photodynamic therapy using meso tetra hydroxy phenyl chlorin (mTHPC) in early prostate cancer. *Lasers Surg Med* 2006;38(5): 356–363

14.

15. Johansson A, et al. Realtime light dosimetry software tools for interstitial photodynamic therapy of the human prostate. *Med Phys* 2007;34(11): 4309–4321.

16. Arumainayagam N, Moore CM, Ahmed HU, Emberton M. Photodynamic therapy for focal ablation of the prostate. *World J Urol* 2010;28(5): 571–576.

CHAPTER 14

Focal Therapy for Prostate Cancer Using Radiation

Irving Kaplan MD[1,2], Elizabeth M. Genega MD[1,2], and Neil Rofsky MD[3]

[1] Beth Israel Deaconess Medical Center, Boston, MA, USA
[2] Harvard Medical School, Boston, MA, USA
[3] Department of Radiology, Beth Israel Deaconess Medical Center, Boston, MA, USA

Introduction

The most common therapeutic approaches for localized prostate cancer include active surveillance or immediate treatment. The role of active surveillance has been reported in several single institutional series but is still being evaluated in the cooperative study setting. The outcomes of these studies are many years in the future. Patients who decide on definitive therapy have multiple options. Radiation options include permanent low dose brachytherapy, high dose rate brachytherapy, standard fractionated external beam irradiation, and accelerated hypofractionated external beam irradiation. These definitive therapies involve treatment of the entire prostate, either removal of the prostate or whole-organ irradiation.

Each of these definitive therapies is associated with short-term and long-term toxicities. In a multi-institution prospective trial using self-reported quality-of-life assessment tools, prostatectomy, external beam irradiation, and brachytherapy, where each associated with a unique pattern of side effects. These side effects impacted on patient's satisfaction and quality of life. Bowel, bladder, and sexual function can be significantly impacted with these therapies [1].

It is important to understand the pathology of prostate cancer to define the appropriate patients for focal therapy. Patients with a single focus of prostate cancer are ideal candidates for focal therapy. However, the majority of men have multifocal disease with small secondary tumors. Determining the accurate location, extent, and grade of the index lesion is

Focal Therapy in Prostate Cancer, First Edition. Edited by Hashim U Ahmed, Manit Arya, Peter Carroll and Mark Emberton.
© 2012 Blackwell Publishing Ltd. Published 2012 by Blackwell Publishing Ltd.

critical in defining which patients are appropriate for focal therapy. The standard selective random biopsy is not adequate.

The size of the index lesion has been found to predict for failure, while the number of small nonindex lesions does not, as discussed in Chapter 3. Furthermore, it is the grade and size of the index lesion that determine clinical outcome after prostatectomy. Small cancers tend to be multifocal bilobar and occur in both peripheral and transitional zone. Focal therapies may not be able to address all these lesions. Therefore, the goal of focal therapy in most patients is not to ablate all foci of cancer but to eradicate the index lesion. The remaining small cancers may not be clinically significant given their low grade and slow growth.

Brachytherapy

Brachytherapy is the placement of radioactivity in or near tumors. It is the oldest form of radiation dating back over 100 years when radium needles where placed into tumors. The use of brachytherapy to treat prostate cancer was first reported in the 1920s by Pasteau and Degrais. Radium needles where applied to the prostate using a transurethral catheter [2].

There are two forms of brachytherapy used to treat prostate cancer: (1) low dose rate (LDR) and (2) high dose rate (HDR) brachytherapy. LDR-brachytherapy entails the permanent placement of radioactive into the prostate. The isotope that is within the sealed source decays over weeks to months delivering radiation. Isotopes that have relatively short half-lives and emit low-energy X-rays are used. Two isotopes are commonly used: (1) iodine-125, which emits 27 KeV X-rays with a half-life of 60 days, and (2) palladium-103, which emits 21 KeV X-rays with a half-life of 17 days.

With HDR-brachytherapy small catheters are placed into the prostate using a transperineal route. A treatment consists of a single highly radioactive iridium-192 source that is transported into the catheters and dwells for specific times and positions within the catheters. Several treatments are delivered several hours apart before the catheters are removed. 192-Iridium emits 0.37 MeV photons.

The clinical utility of brachytherapy is due to the rapid dose fall-off from the source. The combination of attenuation of dose within tissue and geometric dose fall-off from the source (1/distance squared) that leads to 90% of the dose being deposited within 1.0 cm of the source. Partial or focal therapy to only a portion of the prostate with brachytherapy is possible due to the high dose delivery in a small volume of tissue. Using an intraoperative MRI, the group at the Brigham and Women's Hospital performed focal LDR-brachytherapy. On the basis of the low incidence of cancer found in the transition zone in low-risk patients, the peripheral zone and apex alone were the target volume of the implant. Patients with PSA less than 10 ng/mL with Gleason score of 3+4 or less (without perineural invasion) and no palpable disease were eligible for this approach. There was no significant difference in biochemical freedom from relapse in the brachytherapy group when compared to a contemporaneous cohort of men who had undergone radical prostatectomy. The 5-year biochemical control was 93% in the men treated with this approach versus 95% in patients managed with radical prostatectomy [3]. Late genitourinary toxicities were rare, as one would expect given the urethral sparing that was achieved with peripheral-zone targeting [4]. This method of implantation demonstrates that excellent cancer control with low rates of toxicity can be achieved by targeting the peripheral zone and apex in a select group of low-risk men.

Locally recurrent prostate cancer after definitive external beam radiation therapy is unusual occurring in 2–6% of patients [5]. Multiparametric MRI is able to define the area of local failure accurately, with many failures tending to be unifocal (Figure 14.1). Full dose reirradiation of the entire gland is not an option given the unacceptable dose that would be delivered to the rectum and urethra. Focal brachytherapy is a potential salvage strategy for these patients. The group from UCSF reported on 24 patients treated with LDR-brachytherapy after external beam irradiation local failure. Using biopsy information and MR spectroscopy the area of local failure was defined. The target dose to the area of recurrence was full dose (144Gy), while the dose to the entire prostate was reduced to 108Gy. The biochemical relapse free survival was 88% with minimal late rectal and urinary toxicity [6]. Our group at the Beth Israel Deaconess has approached local failure after external beam in a similar fashion. 3T endorectal MRI scans with dynamic contrast enhancement (DCE) are used

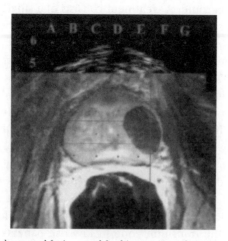

Figure 14.1 MRI-ultrasound fusion used for biopsy. (See Plate 14.1.)

to localize recurrent areas of cancer. After external beam irradiation, the glands are atrophic with slow wash-in and wash-out kinetics, while areas of recurrent cancer demonstrate rapid wash-in and wash-out kinetics. During transperineal biopsy the ultrasound images are fused to the DCE-MRI and used to guide biopsies of suspected and atrophic areas of the prostate [7]. Once histological confirmation is obtained, the patients undergo focal implantation in these areas. In our initial experience of ten patients, all demonstrated rapid PSA declines after focal salvage therapy. With a mean follow-up of 48 months, seven of the ten patients continue to have low stable PSA values [8].

A commonly used mathematic model used to calculate normal and malignant tissue tolerance is the α/β model (based on the linear quadradic fit of the radiation dose survival curve). The numeric value of the α/β ratio is specific for these tissues. Numerous studies have reported that α/β for prostate cancer is approximately 1.5. The α/β for normal tissues is approximately 3. On the basis of the difference of the α/β between prostate cancer and normal tissues, accelerated hypofractionated radiation (high dose per fraction and fewer dose fractions) provides a therapeutic advantage over standard dose fractionation schemes.

As previously discussed, HDR-brachytherapy involves the temporary placement of very high-activity radioactive sources in the prostate administering high dose per fraction radiation treatments. The dose distribution from HDR-brachytherapy is inhomogeneous due to the rapid fall of dose from the center of the radioactive source (1/r2) and the need to keep the rectal and urethral dose below levels that cause toxicity. The dose delivered to the peripheral zone of the prostate is 120–140% of minimum peripheral dose or the prescription dose. In addition, using the α/β model to calculate equivalent total dose, HDR-brachytherapy delivers significantly higher dosage to the prostate than what is achievable with standard external beam techniques. Most commonly, HDR-brachytherapy is used in combination with external beam irradiation. There is an experience using HDR as monotherapy. Table 14.1 reviews the various dose fractionation schemes that have been employed to treat prostate cancer.

Table 14.1 Dose fraction schedules of HDR monotherapy for prostate cancer: biologic equivalents using the α/β model.

Fraction (fx) schedule	Dose/fx	Number of fxs	Total dose	1.5 Gy	3 Gy
Beaumont Hospital HDR [9]	9.5	4	38.0	119.4	95.0
Demanes HDR [10]	7.25	6	43.5	108.8	89.2

Note: All doses expressed in Gy. 2 Gy/fx: biologic equivalent. Assuming an α/β ratio of 1.5 Gy and 3 Gy.

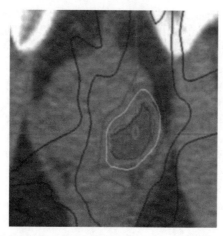

Figure 14.2 Dose distribution using CyberKnife to focally boost radiation dose using MRI to define dominant lesion. (See Plate 14.2.)

External beam irradiation

External beam irradiation can also be used to deliver focal radiation to the prostate. The CyberKnife™ (Accuray, Sunnyvale CA, USA) is a device designed to deliver stereotactic radiation. It utilizes real-time tracking and robotic-controlled radiation delivery to precisely treat small targets. Fuller reported on the feasibility of using CyberKnife to preferentially treat the peripheral zone of the prostate. The entire course of radiation is delivered in four fractions of 9.5Gy [11]. We have treated a select group of patients who have a dominant lesion as demonstrated on endorectal 3T-MRI with a focal boost. The entire prostate is treated to a minimum dose of 7.25Gy for five fractions [12]. The dominant lesion is selectively treated to 120–130% of the prescription dose (Figure 14.2). Long-term follow-up of this dose-painting technique is needed to assess efficacy and toxicities of this approach.

Conclusion

In summary, LDR and HDR brachytherapy and new external beam modalities such as CyberKnife can treat focal areas of the prostate. These forms of radiation can be used to treat only a portion of the prostate or to selectively boost areas within the prostate while minimizing toxicity.

References

1. Sanda MG, et al. Quality of life and satisfaction with outcome among prostate-cancer survivors. *NEJM* 2008;358(12): 1250–1261.

2. Pasteau O, Degrais P. De l'emploi du radium dans letraitementdes cancers de la prostate. *J D'urologie Medicale et Chirurgicale* 1913;4: 341–366.

3. D'amico AV, et al. Comparing PSA outcome after radical prostatectomy or magnetic resonance imaging-guided partial prostatic irradiation in select patients with clinically localized adenocarcinoma of the prostate. *Urology* 2003;62(6): 1063–1067.

4. Albert M, et al. Late genitourinary and gastrointestinal toxicity after magnetic resonance image-guided prostate brachytherapy with or without neoadjuvant external beam radiation therapy. *Cancer* 2003;98(5): 949–954.

5. Kupelian PA, et al. Effect of increasing radiation doses on local and distant failures in patients with localized prostate cancer. *IJROBP* 2008;71(1): 16–22.

6. McKenna DA, et al. Prostate cancer: role of pretreatment MR in predicting outcome after external-beam radiation therapy–initial experience. *Radiology* 2008;247(1): 141–146.

7. Kaplan I, et al. Real time MRI-ultrasound image guided stereotactic prostate biopsy. *Magn Reson Imaging* 2002;20(3): 295–299.

8. Child SK, et al. MRI and ultrasound fusion images to focal guide salvage prostate brachytherapy for local recurrence after external beam radiation therapy: toxicity and outcomes. *ABSTRACT ASCO GU Annual Meeting 2010*.

9. Martinez, et al. Phase II prospective study of the Use of Conformal High-Dose-Rate Brachytherapy as MonoTherapy for the Treatment of Favorable Stage Prstate Cancer: A feasibility Study. *Int J Radiat Oncol Biol Phys* 2001;49(1): 61.

10. Schour, et al. High Dose Rate Monotherapy for Prostate Cancer. *IJROBP* 2005;63(1 Suppl): S315.

11. Fuller DB, et al. Virtual HDR CyberKnife treatment for localized prostatic carcinoma: dosimetry comparison with HDR brachytherapy and preliminary clinical observations. *IJROBP* 2008;70(5): 1588–1597.

12. King CR, et al. Stereotactic body radiotherapy for localized prostate cancer: interim results of a prospective phase II clinical trial. *IJROBP* 2009;73(4): 1043–1048.

CHAPTER 15

Image Registration and Fusion for Image-Guided Focal Ablation

Dean C. Barratt PhD and David J. Hawkes PhD CPhys FMedSci FREng FInstP FIPEM

UCL Centre for Medical Image Computing, University College London, London, UK

Introduction

Image registration—the process of aligning images—is an important prerequisite for implementing focal ablation strategies, since it allows a treatment plan based on data obtained prior to an intervention to be spatially related to transrectal ultrasound (TRUS) images obtained during the intervention. In practice, such a treatment plan contains precise information on the location and extent of target tumors determined by biopsy mapping, magnetic resonance (MR) imaging, or a combination of both. If a three-dimensional representation of a treatment plan can be successfully registered to TRUS images, it can be presented as an overlay to aid surgical navigation (Figure 15.1). However, deformation of the prostate and the need for high accuracy and minimal user interaction in order to ensure minimal disruption to the normal clinical workflow present significant technical challenges. The need for high accuracy is particularly acute for focal therapy since accurate treatment delivery to one or more well-defined target regions is a fundamental prerequisite to achieving optimal therapeutic effect while minimizing the risk of treatment-related complications. Image registration also plays an important role in registering posttreatment images with pretreatment images (or an associated treatment plan) in order to assess treatment efficacy by comparing regions of necrosis or suspected residual/recurrent cancer against the desired ablation.

Registration versus fusion

The terms *image fusion* and *image registration* are often used interchangeably, particularly in clinical circles, but for the purposes of this discussion,

Focal Therapy in Prostate Cancer, First Edition. Edited by Hashim U Ahmed, Manit Arya, Peter Carroll and Mark Emberton.

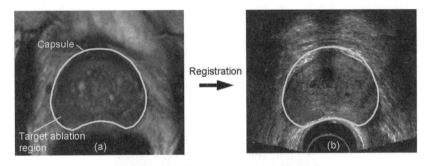

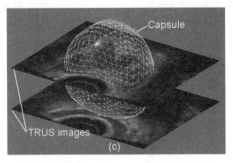

Figure 15.1 (a) A slice through a T2-weighted MR volume of the prostate with a target region for focal ablation shown in red. (b) Registered TRUS image with the MR-derived therapy plan overlaid. (c) Three-dimensional representation of an MR-derived therapy plan registered with a TRUS image volume (only two slices of this volume are shown for clarity). Once registered, the therapy plan can be used in conjunction with intraoperative TRUS images to aid precise therapy delivery. (See Plate 15.1.)

it is instructive to note the following technical distinction: image fusion refers to the process of combining multiple sources of image data into a single representation. Therefore, the image fusion process is largely concerned with the visual representation of multiple sources of (coregistered) image data as a single image, which is a significantly more concise representation of the input data and lends itself to easier visual interpretation and analysis. Importantly, image fusion algorithms enable different sources of data to be weighted according to their importance or relevance for a particular task prior to the final presentation. For example, sites of low-risk disease are omitted from the representation illustrated in Figure 15.1, since they do not form part of the *treatment* plan. Image registration on the other hand refers to the process of transforming multiple images into a common coordinate system, which is a prerequisite task for image fusion. Therefore, images must be registered before they can be fused. In the remainder of this chapter, the emphasis is on image registration as a means to achieving image fusion.

Practical aspects of image registration

In practice, image registration involves determining the mathematical transformation that maps the location of each pixel or voxel (volumetric element—a three-dimensional pixel) in one image to a corresponding location in a second image. As indicated in Figure 15.2, each image is commonly identified as either the *source* or the *target* image and the transformation (denoted by T) has a direction, such that applying the transformation to the source image results in that image being aligned spatially with the target image. Different transformation models have different *degrees of freedom,* defined as the number of parameters that specify a particular transformation. The problem of determining this transformation is simplified considerably if it is assumed to represent a rigid-body transformation, where only translations and rotations are allowed and therefore the

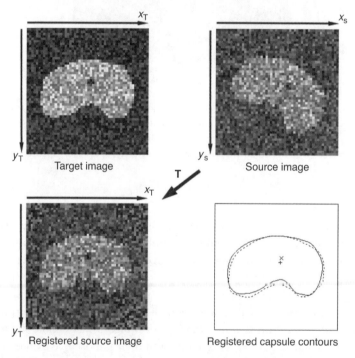

Figure 15.2 Example of the registration of a source image (top right) to a target (or reference) image of a prostate gland (top left). After applying the registration transformation, T, to transform the pixel coordinates of the source image to the target image coordinate system (indicated by the x_T and y_T axes), the transformed source image (bottom left) is aligned with the target image. The bottom right diagram shows the capsule boundaries and urethral locations for the registered images to provide a more precise visual assessment of the registration. (Note: The images presented in this figure are intended for illustrative purposes and do not represent images obtained using any particular imaging modality).

structures represented by the image can move but remain the same shape following transformation (Figure 15.2). For two-dimensional images, a rigid-body transformation has three degrees of freedom (two translations and one rotation), whereas in three-dimensional a rigid-body transformation is described by three translations and three rotations, resulting in six degrees of freedom. Therefore, a rigid registration of two volumetric images will involve determining six parameters that optimally align these images.

Although the assumption of rigidity simplifies the registration problem significantly, its validity very much depends on the application: rigid registration is appropriate for registering bony anatomy, but it may not be appropriate when significant soft-tissue deformation has occurred between imaging sessions. This is a particular problem for conventional neuronavigation systems, which allow accurate registration of the skull, but are subject to significant error in procedures involving a craniotomy since significant brain shift typically occurs. As the prostate gland is a deformable organ, the assumption of rigidity may not be appropriate in the typical case where insertion of a TRUS probe deforms the prostate significantly compared, for instance, to its state as represented by an MR scan. The deformation between MR and TRUS images may be even more pronounced if an endorectal coil is used during MR imaging. Prostate deformation also occurs as a result of changes in patient position (for example, supine versus lithotomy), bladder filling, normal rectal motion, and respiration. During therapy, large deformations are also commonly observed as a result of gland swelling in response to needle injury and tissue ablation.

The propensity of the prostate gland to deform between different imaging time-points indicates that so-called *nonrigid registration* techniques, which compute more complicated transformations with a relatively large number of degrees of freedom, are required to account for deformation and achieve the high level of targeting accuracy demanded by focal therapy. Many such techniques exist [1], but these have the overhead of increased complexity and computational burden compared with rigid registration approaches.

Once an appropriate transformation model has been established, image registration approaches can be broadly classed into two types, sometimes refered to as *feature-* or *intensity*-based methods. In feature-based approach, each image is first processed to extract common "features," which might be fiducial markers, tissue boundaries, or anatomical structures that can be represented geometrically by a point, line, or surface. The process of extracting such features is known as image segmentation and a wide range of software tools now exist for this purpose, ranging from those where features are identified manually by the user to those which exploit sophisticated image analysis techniques to partially or completely automate the task. Once a set of corresponding features has been defined for each input image, the registration transformation can be computed automatically by employing a point, line, or surface matching method.

In the prostate, a straightforward registration method used by some commercial systems is to align the capsule after it has been contoured in each input image. However, it is of most clinical value to register structures inside the gland, principally tumors, which, as noted above, often do not appear in all of the images to be registered. In this case, registration on the basis of matching internal features become problematic. However, even if the registration is nonrigid, it is possible to predict the displacement of internal structures by interpolating pixel/voxel displacements across the gland or by using a physical model of tissue deformation, such as a finite element model (FEM) [2]. The latter has the advantage that taking into account the physics of gland deformation potentially leads to a more accurate prediction of tissue displacement, but building a multicompartment FEM from image data and determining the tissue mechanical properties and boundary conditions associated with a particular motion is a challenging task in practice.

In contrast to feature-based registration, intensity-based approaches attempt to register images using pixel/voxel gray-level (intensity) values alone by maximizing some measure of image similarity, which is a function of these gray-level values. This requires defining a measure of image similarity that takes its maximum value when images are aligned. A large number of similarity measures have been proposed. One of the simplest is to simply sum the square of the difference between adjacent pixel/voxel values in the input values. This measure, called sum-of-squared-differences, is useful for the purposes of illustrating an intensity-based similarity measure, but is seldom used in practice for directly registering images from different modalities (say, a CT and an MR image) because it is not robust to differences in intensity distributions between such images. Information theoretic measures, including entropy-based measures such as mutual information, on the other hand have in general been found to be more accurate for multimodal registration.

In general, intensity-based registration methods have the advantage that performing a registration requires very little or no user interaction, and, unlike feature-based approaches, do not require prior feature segmentation. Automatic alternatives to feature-based registration methods are especially important for time-critical, surgical applications where software tools to segment intraoperative images are either not available, not sufficiently reliable, or too time-consuming or difficult to use to be clinically practical.

Recently, a number of automatic and semiautomatic (i.e., those requiring a reasonable level of manual interaction) techniques have emerged for segmenting the capsule in prostate ultrasound and MR images [3–6]. However, these have yet to be widely adopted and, since ultrasound images are subject to a range of artifacts and have relatively poor and variable quality, manual contouring remains the most reliable and accurate method used in clinical practice. Consequently, feature-based registration approaches typically incur a significant time overhead to segment the capsule (and in some cases additional structures, such as the urethra).

Application to prostate biopsy and interventions

Several research groups have investigated deformable methods for registering MR images of the prostate acquired at different times, with or without the use of an endorectal coil. Crouch et al. [7] describe a method for automatically generating a computer model of the prostate gland, using FEM techniques, and using this to register CT and TRUS images obtained with and without an MR endorectal coil in place. Interestingly, their method also compensates for the effect of gland swelling following brachytherapy seed implantation.

Methods for registering MR and TRUS images are also described. Singh et al. [8] describe a manual method for nonrigidly registering MR and TRUS images, but this requires significant user interaction during a procedure to align both the capsule and structures inside the prostate. An automatic registration technique, reported by Wu et al. [9], adopts a novel "marker-to-pixel" approach in which the prostate capsule surface (the "marker"), segmented from one three-dimensional TRUS image, is rigidly registered directly to another TRUS image of the same patient. Further work by Shao et al. [10] investigated methods for registering the pubic arch in MR and TRUS images, comparing the similarity measure proposed by Wu et al. with alternative measures. Results were presented for the accuracy of registering the pubic arch, but unfortunately the registration error was not reported for the prostate gland.

Most recently, algorithms for registering TRUS images, acquired at different time-points during a procedure, have been reported [11]. By combining such a method with an initial registration of an MR image and TRUS images, obtained at the start of the procedure, the transformation between the MR image and each subsequent set of TRUS images can be determined and the registration updated during the course of a procedure. The same approach can be used to register a biopsy plan, which is updated to account for deformation due to movement of the TRUS probe, for example. A recent study by Xu et al. [12] demonstrates the application of a method for MR-to-TRUS registration during freehand transrectal biopsy using an end-firing TRUS probe. Using CT imaging to identify needle tip locations, the accuracy of the system in localizing the centers for target tumors within a prostate phantom was reported to be 2.4 ± 1.2 mm. A further evaluation of the registration accuracy on the basis of the overlap between capsule contours drawn on two-dimensional MR and TRUS images selected from 20 patient datasets yielded a $90 \pm 7\%$ following registration. However, no data were provided on the accuracy of registering internal anatomy of the gland and the registration assumes that the prostate gland moves as a rigid, nondeformable structure. Furthermore, an initial (manual) registration of the MR and TRUS images is required at the start of a procedure, but details of this process are not provided.

An alternative registration approach adopts the general framework in which a biomechanical model of soft-tissue deformation is used to provide training data for a statistical model of organ motion, which can be used to predict the motion of the prostate gland under different (boundary) conditions, which correspond to different positions and orientations of the TRUS probe, for example. Hu et al. [13] describe the application of this method for generating a biomechanically constrained deformable model of the prostate gland. In another report the authors present a novel "model-to-image" registration method, which allows automatic registration of the deformable prostate model surface to the TRUS images. Validation of the method using matched MR and three-dimensional TRUS datasets obtained on seven patients yielded a mean target registration error, on the basis of intracapsular landmarks, such as cysts and the urethra, of 2.36 mm [14].

Accuracy validation

In keeping with the best clinical and scientific practice, it is extremely important to properly validate the accuracy of image registration methods in as realistic a setting as possible. This can be challenging, as it is often difficult to establish a sufficiently accurate gold standard in vivo against which a new registration algorithm may be compared. A number of error measures have been devised for evaluating registration accuracy. The simplest method is visual inspection of how well-aligned images are, but this is highly subjective and does not achieve the precision provided by quantitative methods that is required to rigorously compare different registrations. A popular method, which does not suffer from these limitations, is to measure the distance between corresponding anatomical or fiducial landmarks following registration. To avoid bias, landmarks should be identified independently in each image and, for feature-based registration methods in particular, should not coincide with the features used to perform the registration, since the algorithm will attempt to minimize this distance and therefore this error measure may be unrepresentative of errors in regions away from the landmarks. Furthermore, to ensure that error measures are most useful, landmarks should define "targets" that are located in positions highly relevant to the clinical application. In this case, the distance errors are commonly referred as *target registration errors* (TREs). Computing TREs on the basis of identifiable landmarks can be challenging in practice, since often the anatomical structures that are of most clinical interest are only visible on one of the images, as is the case for TRUS and MR images of the prostate. However, it is usually possible to identify alternative landmarks, such as cysts and calcifications (Figure 15.3).

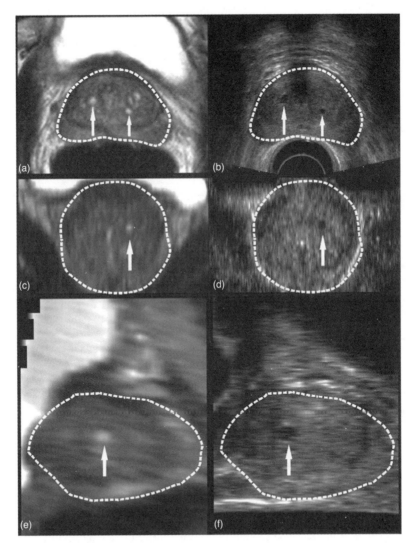

Figure 15.3 Orthogonal views through registered MR (left: (a), (c), (d)) and TRUS (right: (b), (d), (f)) images; from top to bottom: transverse (a,b), coronal (c,d), and sagittal views (e,f) of the prostate gland. The arrows indicate corresponding anatomical landmarks (cysts in this case) that can be used to calculate target registration errors (TREs) in order to quantify registration accuracy.

Future work

Registration of a treatment plan to intraoperative TRUS (or MR) images is technically identical to the problem of registering a biopsy plan or a population-based cancer atlas. Therefore, work in this area is highly relevant to focal therapy applications, particularly as biopsy data currently forms an important part of the information used to construct a treatment plan. Moreover, several dedicated three-dimensional ultrasound-guided biopsy systems are now commercially available, which provide more accurate localization of tissue samples than conventional TRUS-guided biopsy. Registration of this information with image-based data for the purposes of directing therapy is an important task for focal therapy applications. Since the most recent evidence suggests that multiparametric MR appears to provide the most accurate means of localizing prostate cancer, registration of different MR images is an additional important task for meaningful interpretation of information provided by multiple sequences, for example, by computer-aided diagnosis.

References

1. Hajnal JV, et al. *Medical Image Registration*. CRC Press, Boca Raton, FL; 2001.
2. Carter TJ, et al. Application of soft tissue modelling to image-guided surgery. *Med Eng Phys* 2005;27(10): 893–909.
3. Betrouni N, et al. 3D delineation of prostate, rectum and bladder on MR images. *Comput Med Imaging Graph* 2008;32(7): 622–630.
4. Cool D, et al. 3D prostate model formation from non-parallel 2D ultrasound biopsy images. *Med Image Anal* 2006;10(6): 875–887.
5. Hodge AC, et al. Prostate boundary segmentation from ultrasound images using 2D active shape models: optimisation and extension to 3D. *Comput Methods Programs Biomed* 2006;84(2–3): 99–113.
6. Klein S, et al. Automatic segmentation of the prostate in 3D MR images by atlas matching using localized mutual information. *Med Phys* 2008;35(4): 1407–1417.
7. Crouch JR, et al. Automated finite-element analysis for deformable registration of prostate images. *IEEE Trans Med Imag* 2007;26(10): 1379–1390.
8. Singh AK, et al. Initial clinical experience with real-time transrectal ultrasonography-magnetic resonance imaging fusion-guided prostate biopsy. *BJUInt* 2008;101(7): 841–845.
9. Wu R, et al. Registration of organ surface with intra-operative ultrasound image using genetic algorithm. *Medical Image Computing and Computer-Assisted Intervention – MICCAI 2003*. LNCS 2878 ed. Springer, Berlin; 2003. pp. 383–390.
10. Shao W, et al. Evaluation on similarity measures of a surface-to-image registration technique for ultrasound images. *Medical Image Computing and Computer-Assisted Intervention – MICCAI 2006*. LNCS 4191 ed. Springer, Berlin; 2006. pp. 742–749.
11. Baumann M, et al. *Prostate biopsy assistance system with gland deformation estimation for enhanced precision*. MICCAI 2009. LNCS 5761 (Part 1). Springer, Berlin; 2009. pp. 67–74.

12. Xu S, et al. Real-time MRI-TRUS fusion for guidance of targeted prostate biopsies. *Computer Aided Surgery* 2008;13(5): 255–264.
13. Hu Y, et al. Modelling prostate gland motion for image-guided interventions. *Biomedical Simulation*. LNCS 5104 ed. Springer, Berlin; 2008. pp. 79–88.
14. Hu Y, et al. *MR to ultrasound image registration for guiding prostate biopsy and interventions*. MICCAI 2009. LNCS 5761 (Part 1). Springer, Berlin; 2009. pp. 787–794.

SECTION IV

How can we determine the success of Focal Therapy?

CHAPTER 16

Determining Success of Focal Therapy: Biochemical and Biopsy Strategies

Al B. Barqawi MD FRCS[1], Paul D. Maroni MD[2], and E. David Crawford MD[3]

[1] Division of Urology, University of Colorado Denver School of Medicine, Aurora, CO, USA
[2] Division of Urology, Department of Surgery, University of Colorado School of Medicine, Aurora, CO, USA
[3] University of Colorado, Denver, Aurora, CO, USA

Introduction

Clinical centers performing targeted treatments have developed arbitrarily algorithms for assessing success on the basis of their own experience, and currently no consensus exists among treating physicians on the ultimate guidelines [1,2] (Table 16.1). Ensuring oncologic control after focal treatment of prostate malignancies becomes problematic given the current methods of monitoring and detecting cancer recurrence. PSA is the most widely used marker and, in fact, is the only item used for following patients after treatment in most standard clinical practice circumstances. History, physical, other laboratory testing, and radiologic testing using current techniques and methods reveal surprisingly little prior to an increase in the PSA level. Definitions of biochemical recurrence are abundant but are in some cases controversial. Those biochemical definitions that are validated within existing practice for whole-gland therapies should be applied carefully in the setting of focal therapy until treatment processes are standardized and outcomes are better defined. Follow-up schedules from active surveillance protocols would be the more sensible approach to monitoring oncologic efficacy after focal treatment, but the validity of these for surveillance have come into question.

Focal Therapy in Prostate Cancer, First Edition. Edited by Hashim U Ahmed, Manit Arya, Peter Carroll and Mark Emberton.
© 2012 Blackwell Publishing Ltd. Published 2012 by Blackwell Publishing Ltd.

Table 16.1 Follow-up protocols in focal treatment and active surveillance trials.

Management	Series	Clinical	PSA	Biopsy
Focal	Bahn et al. [3]		q3 months	6, 12, 24, and 60 months or with PSA progression
	Ellis et al. [4]		q3 months for 1 year, then q6 months	
	Lambert et al. [5]	3, 6, and 12 months, then q6 months	3, 6, and 12 months, then q6 months	With PSA progression
	Onik et al. [7]		q3 months for 2 years, then q6 months	At 12 months or with PSA progression
	Muto et al. [6]			
	Ahmed et al.		q3 months for 1 year, then q6 months	Multiparametric MRI if PSA progression, then biopsy (either transperineal template or TRUS dependent on MRI)
Active surveillance	Toronto		q3 months × 2 years, then q6 months	6–12 months after diagnosis then every 3–4 years
	Johns Hopkins	q6 months	q6 months	Annual

Defining biochemical recurrence

In focal therapy, the proportion of tissue ablated varies widely as a result of differences in the location, volume, and cancer grade. Therefore, the expected PSA levels in such cases are variable and not only reflect the volume of the residual prostate gland (PSA density), but may also be significantly influenced by the following factors:

1 The proportion of preoperative PSA that is specific to the cancer diagnosis.
2 The accuracy of the targeted ablation technique.
3 The presence of and rate of natural progression of benign prostatic hyperplasia (BPH).
4 The presence of inflammation and the timing of its onset.
5 The use of 5-alpha reductase inhibitors, pre- and postoperatively.

Due to these factors, an ideal PSA nadir level, therefore, is unpredictable following focal therapy. PSA does tend to decrease after focal treatment by 30–60% [3–7]. In the Colorado series of 60 men treated with targeted focal cryotherapy for localized prostate cancer, the mean PSA value at 3 months was 50% lower than preoperative PSA. In a trial using high-intensity focused ultrasound to ablate unilateral cancer, the PSA decreased by approximately 80% at 6 months [8]. The best definition to determine biochemical recurrence after focal treatment is unknown. A specific threshold for PSA nadir would have poor predictive value given the wide range of PSA levels observed after successful focal treatment. Given a detectable PSA occurs by nature, many groups have used the ASTRO criteria (three rises from nadir) as a definition of biochemical recurrence. The rationale for this is relatively sound; patients after radiation or focal treatment have detectable PSAs that might be due to residual cancer and PSA kinetics matter. A more rapidly rising PSA may not only be indicative of residual cancer, but biologically aggressive cancer that would require retreatment. The ASTRO definition is also easy to use and identifiable.

Biochemical disease free status (bDFS) using ASTRO criteria ranges between 80% and 93%. Time to failure determinations are inconsistently published, but these data seem to be for periods of at least 2 years. Onik et al. included retreatment patients in the bDFS calculation and the success of a single treatment was reduced at 85% (7 of 48 patients failed) from 94% [5]. It is notable that only 23 of 48 patients in this study were low-risk patients (PSA <10 ng/dL, ≤T2a, Gleason ≤6). Results in low- versus intermediate- and high-risk patients were not presented. Lambert et al. used a bDFS definition of not achieving a ≥50% decrease in PSA and reported an 84% recurrence-free survival; however, few patients had a repeat prostate biopsy [3]. The focal treatment approaches and procedures were variable. Treatment targeted at cancer-containing areas was used in some studies and planned hemiablation was used in others.

Radiation oncologists have migrated nearly completely to the Phoenix definition (PSA nadir + 2). The argument for not using the Phoenix definition for defining disease recurrence after focal treatments is more angular. Radiation treatments are expected to ablate all or nearly all of the prostate gland and nadirs are expected to be very low (PSA <1 ng/dL). This has been repeatedly observed over the past several decades. The Phoenix definition is felt to be very specific for disease recurrence in patients after radiation treatment. Only one study presented recurrence data using the Phoenix definition and the bDFS was 88% with 28 months median follow-up [3].

Focal treatments leave substantial portions of the prostate gland intact (Figure 16.1) and PSA nadirs are not nearly as low. Mean PSA levels after focal treatment are between 2 ng/dL and 3 ng/dL. In untreated prostate

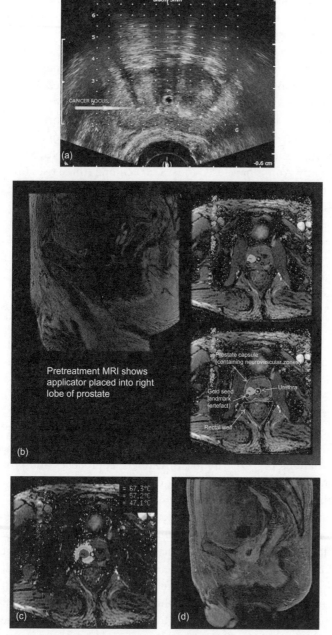

Figure 16.1   Series of figures demonstrating a focal therapy using an interstitial photothermal ablative therapy with an in-bore MRI. Template-mapping biopsies located the cancer in the right lobe of the prostate (a); the applicator was placed accurately into this area during treatment and verified on MRI (b); real-time feedback using MRI thermometry is possible to ensure adequate ablation limited to the targeted area (c); early verification using a postgadolinium contrast MRI demonstrating perfusion deficit in the treated area (d). (See Plate 16.1.)

glands peculiar and temporary rises of the PSA by several points for entirely benign reasons are common. Likewise, patients on active surveillance have some variability in the PSA suggesting that rises are not always explained by cancer progression. A repeated rise over three PSA examinations is felt to be less likely to occur in the absence of active cancer. Also at issue is the impact of BPH progression in residual tissue and use of 5-alpha reductase inhibitors. The University of Colorado targeted treatment protocol recommends the use of dutasteride in all patients following focal lesion ablation. In addition to control of BPH-related PSA rises, we feel there is a benefit of primary and/or secondary cancer prevention in this population. This hypothesis is based on the observed effects of 5-ARIs in primary prevention trials. For biochemical follow-up, we recommend PSA checks every 4 months for the first 2 years, then biannually. Mandatory interval prostate biopsy should be required in any patient receiving focal treatment to help develop a clear and usable definition of biochemical recurrence.

Determining histological local recurrence

The repeat prostate biopsy presents challenges that can prevent science and a pragmatic approach necessary in clinical practice from meeting. To prove oncologic efficacy, diagnostic accuracy is critical. In a 2007 statement by an international task force, "outcome measures for focal therapy trials should at a minimum include...extensive post-treatment biopsy mapping to determine treatment effect and identify disease persistence" [9]. Currently, the most accurate biopsy techniques are the most cumbersome and expensive. While straightforward, transrectal biopsies commonly understage and undergrade cancers. Recent articles have also highlighted worries that repeated transrectal prostate biopsies are not as innocuous as commonly perceived; more numerous prostate biopsies with time seem to have a direct relationship with the development of sexual dysfunction. Since a primary goal of focal treatments is to minimize side effects, a repeat prostate biopsy may create a burden of survivorship contrary to this end.

If PSA kinetics suggests biologically active disease and a routine TRUS biopsy is negative, a transperineal template-mapping biopsy should be strongly considered. Assuming thorough pretreatment biopsy was performed and revealed low-volume, low- or intermediate-risk disease, disseminated disease would be unlikely and an assiduous search for local disease should be carried out. Imaging with multiparametric MRI is another alternative and will be discussed in Chapter 16.

Several studies of focal treatment had posttreatment biopsies designed in the follow-up plan. Compliance with follow-up prostate biopsy ranged from 50% to 86% and positive prostate biopsies were seen in 4–40%.

Positive prostate biopsies were almost universally from untreated parts of the prostate gland. Studies utilizing either a transperineal template biopsy scheme or Doppler ultrasound to identify contralateral cancer prior to focal treatment had lower rates of positive posttreatment histology. This highlights the need for careful patient selection, as patients with disease in untreated parts of the prostate likely had this cancer present at diagnosis [10–12]. Numerous studies only recommend repeat prostate biopsy if certain PSA criteria were met, although this incorporates a significant work-up bias detrimental to developing robust biochemical measures of failure.

Patients with disease recurrence or disease persistence in the cryoablation studies were almost universally retreated with the same modality. Repeat cryoablation was able to salvage 66–100% of patients with documented local recurrences. Retreatment in the one HIFU study consisted of androgen deprivation therapy, but this study generally had higher risk patients [4]. The one prospective trial published using HIFU showed absence of clinically significant cancer in the treated areas of all men biopsied, but two men had 1 mm of Gleason 6 disease; one of these opted for retreatment and the other surveillance [6]. Information about salvage procedures other than repeat ablation after focal therapy is lacking.

Until optimal targeted prostate cancer treatment techniques are established, mandatory repeat transrectal 12-core biopsy should be performed at years 1, 3, and 5 and at PSA progression. In our experience with salvage prostatectomy after focal treatment in one patient, marked fibrosis was noted on the side of treatment, but the contralateral side seemed unaffected. Without more information about the ability to perform salvage procedures successfully and with low morbidity, patients should be counseled prefocal therapy regarding the potential for this treatment to impact future treatment alternatives.

Creating a responsible and pragmatic follow-up strategy

The primary goal of follow-up should be the prompt detection of clinically significant persistent or recurrent prostate cancer. While new biological recurrence markers should be investigated, PSA and repeat biopsy will be the cornerstones of detection of disease. Follow-up should also be stratified by risk. If patients were low-risk at diagnosis, follow-up strategies similar to active surveillance protocols seem to be the most sensible. Similarly, this may be reasonable in older patients or patients with limited life expectancy and higher risk disease. Low-risk protocols typically recommend PSA checks at 3–6 months intervals with repeat biopsies every 1–3 years. Follow-up end points that would usually result in a recommendation to choose treatment are grade progression on biopsy, an increase in the volume of cancer present, or a PSA doubling time of less than 3 years. PSA kinetics alone should not indicate whole-gland treatment without pathologic confirmation of recurrent or persistent cancer. Distant disease should be ruled out. If a transrectal biopsy is negative and there is still concern for residual local disease, a thorough transperineal biopsy to sample anterior and apical areas of the prostate gland should be strongly considered.

Our current practice is to measure serum PSA and perform rectal examination at 3-month intervals for the first 2 years and every 6 months thereafter following targeted focal therapy (TFT). All patients undergo standard 12-core transrectal biopsy at 1 year after treatment. In addition, an earlier rebiopsy is considered in the setting of an increasing PSA to a value greater than pretreatment PSA, a short PSA doubling time (<24 months), and a change in rectal examination findings. In patients with borderline increases in PSA, other biomarkers that have been found to have utility in the prediagnostic setting such as urinary PCA3 test may be indicated. The clinical utility of urinary and serum biomarkers in follow-up after focal therapy requires robust validation in clinical trials.

Conclusion

In summary, the ideal definition for biochemical recurrence has yet to be determined. Both ASTRO and Phoenix criteria could be used to identify cancer recurrence and may be used to trigger repeat prostate biopsy. Routine repeat prostate biopsy of treated and untreated parts of the prostate should be strongly considered. If local recurrence is detected and distant disease is ruled out, cancer and patient factors should be taken into account to determine the best treatment plan. Retreatment with ablation has the added value of being able to salvage most local failures without resorting to whole-gland surgery or radiotherapy.

In this era with a focus on clinical outcomes and evidence-based medicine, treatments for prostate cancer will need to meet concrete oncologic and functional endpoints. Focal prostate cancer treatments need to prove that they are more than a costly placebo. They will need to show minimization of treatment-related morbidity and durable control of local disease. A careful eye will also be cast on the costs of treatment and the burden of survivorship. The performance of randomized trials proving noninferiority of focal treatments to other modalities seems unlikely, but should still be considered using pragmatic designs that fit with existing clinical equipoise in order to maximize recruitment [13]. Success may be measured in many ways, but those providing focal treatments should strive for a cost-effective, low-impact procedure that allows the patient to die of other causes without suffering from local or distant prostate cancer.

Acknowledgment

Joseph Dallera, MD assisted with preparation of brief portions of the manuscript.

References

1. Ahmed HU, et al. Focal therapy in prostate cancer: determinants of success and failure. *J Endourol* 2010;24(5): 819–825.
2. Ahmed HU, Emberton M. Benchmarks for success in focal therapy of prostate cancer: cure or control? *World J Urol* 2010;28(5): 577–582.
3. Bahn DK, et al. Focal Prostate Cryoablation: Initial Results Show Cancer Control and Potency Preservation. *J Endourol* 2006;20(9): 688–692.
4. Ellis DS, et al. Focal Cryosurgery Followed by Penile Rehabilitation as Primary Treatment for Localized Prostate Cancer: Initial Results. *Urology* 2007;70(Suppl 6A): 9–15.
5. Lambert EH, et al. Focal Cryosurgery: Encouraging health outcomes for unifocal prostate cancer. *Urology* 2007;69: 1117–1120.
6. Muto S, et al. Focal Therapy with High-intensity-focused ultrasound in the treatment of localized prostate cancer. *Jpn J Clinical Oncol* 2008;38(3): 192–199.
7. Onik G, et al. The "male lumpectomy": Focal therapy for prostate cancer using cryoablation results in 48 patients with at least 2-year follow-up. *Urol Oncol* 2008;26: 500–505.
8. Ahmed HU et al. Focal Therapy in men with localised prostate cancer: a phase I/II trial. *J Urol* 2011;185(4): 1246–1254..
9. Eggener SE, et al. Focal therapy for localized prostate cancer: a critical appraisal of rationale and modalities. *J Urol* 2007;178: 2260–2267.
10. Tareen B, et al. Laterality alone should not drive selection of candidates for hemi-ablative focal therapy. *J Urol* 2009;181: 1082–1090.
11. Polascik TJ, et al. Patient selection for hemiablative focal therapy of prostate cancer. *Cancer* 2009;115: 2104–2110.
12. Falzarano SM, et al. Can saturation biopsy predict prostate cancer localization in radical prostatectomy specimens: a correlative study and implications for focal therapy. *Urology* 2010;76(3): 682–687.
13. Crawford ED, Tangen CM. Clinical trials: 'clinical integration': laudable, but challenging. *Nat Rev Urol* 2009;6(6): 297–298.

CHAPTER 17

Determining Success of Focal Therapy: Imaging

Alex Kirkham FRCR MD BM BCh FRCS and Clare Allen FRCR MD BM BCh

Department of Radiology, University College Hospital NHS Foundation Trust, London, UK

Introduction

There are several ways of defining success. The international working group on image-guided tumor ablation makes an important distinction between "technical success," "technique effectiveness," and outcome [1]. *Technical success* is a measure of whether the tumor, in any given session, was treated according to protocol and covered completely, and is mainly the result of correct targeting and adequate treatment intensity. *Technique effectiveness* refers to the absence of tumor at a predetermined point of clinical follow-up. *Outcome* is primarily a clinical measure, but imaging follow-up is an important predictor, particularly in the prostate where low-grade, low-volume tumors may take decades to become clinically apparent.

We will divide this chapter into three sections, corresponding to the use of imaging at three different points after the delivery of focal treatment. The first is during treatment, to confirm that the therapy has been targeted and delivered at the correct intensity, and might be termed *real-time feedback*. The second is soon after treatment, when after ablative techniques we are in a position to assess necrosis, although it may also be possible to detect residual tumor. A scan at this point may provide valuable information to the operator to refine their technique, and prognostic information for the patient: we might call it "quality assurance" or treatment *verification*. Finally, we must be in a position to detect residual or recurrent disease, and the final section of the chapter will address *follow-up*.

To some extent, we will address the techniques used for focal therapy as a group, but there are important differences. Ablation (by heat or cold) produces almost immediate coagulative necrosis, whereas in

Focal Therapy in Prostate Cancer, First Edition. Edited by Hashim U Ahmed, Manit Arya, Peter Carroll and Mark Emberton.

© 2012 Blackwell Publishing Ltd. Published 2012 by Blackwell Publishing Ltd.

photodynamic therapy and in particular radiotherapy it may be hours, days, or months before the effects of treatment are maximal. In addition, the tissue response to salvage treatment (if there has been previous radiotherapy) is considerably different to the naive gland. Finally, the field is young, and the number of publications on imaging follow-up after focal therapy is still in single figures: extrapolation of many of the studies for the whole prostate will be necessary, and (a common refrain) much more research is needed.

Real-time feedback in ablative techniques

Although ultrasound cannot yet be used for accurate thermometry, it can be used for real-time monitoring of ablation in several ways. In cryotherapy, the edge of the ice ball near the probe is distinct, and in HIFU there are gray scale hyperechoic (deemed "Uchida") changes due to cavitation and boiling. In radio-frequency ablation or microwave treatment, microbubbles are seen at the edge of the treated zone, and in brachytherapy ultrasound can be used to confirm seed placement or needle position. Ultrasound can also be used to assess vascularity, particularly when intravenous enhancement is used, and has been used to demonstrate the growing perfusion defect during laser thermotherapy [2] (Figure 17.1).

A potentially more elegant method of feedback is in the use of thermometry, particularly in thermoablation, and it is here that MRI has the potential to provide real-time measurement of heating and a feedback loop that ensures temperature sufficient for cell kill in the treated volume. There are several parameters on MR that vary with temperature, including spin-lattice relaxation time (T1), proton resonance frequency (spectroscopy), and diffusion. With these techniques spatial resolution of 1 mm, temperature resolution of $2°C$, and scan times of the order of a second can be achieved, although there is an inevitable trade-off between the parameters. Furthermore, it is easier to measure *change* in temperature than its absolute value. One commercial system that makes use of real-time proton diffusion-based thermometry in a closed loop to modulate the intensity of HIFU energy delivery is available and has shown promise in the treatment of fibroids. Similar systems are under development for the prostate, but inferring absolute temperature becomes less reliable when rectal cooling is added to the equation, producing an unpredictable posterior temperature gradient.

Thermometry of frozen tissue is possible in the prostate using $R2^*$-weighted imaging and has been demonstrated in dogs, although the resolution is of the order of several millimeters. However, the most effective use of MRI in cryotherapy is currently the delineation of the ice ball, which

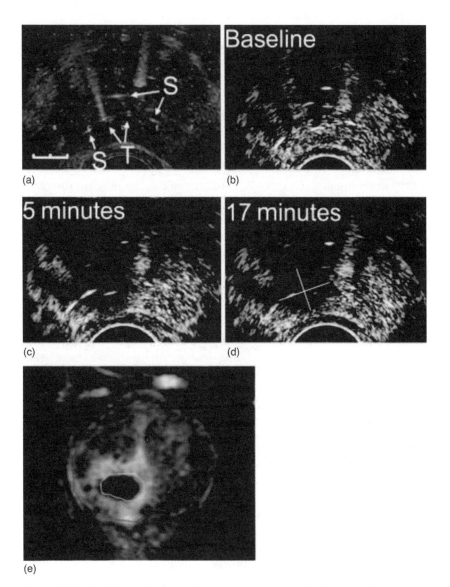

Figure 17.1 Evolving perfusion defect on contrast-enhanced ultrasound during interstitial laser thermotherapy. (a) A transverse ultrasound image for treatment planning. T marks treatment fibers and S sensory fibers. (b–d) Contrast-enhanced (0.2 mL Definity, Lantheus Medical Imaging, N. Billerica, MA, USA) ultrasound images before and 5 and 17 minutes after the start of treatment. (e) The corresponding contrast-enhanced MRI showing an equivalent defect in enhancement 7 days after treatment. The circle corresponds to the defect seen on ultrasound. (By kind permission of Drs R Weersink, M Gertner, and J Trachtenberg and the *Canadian Urological Association Journal.*) (See Plate 17.1.)

is well seen on T2 sequences as an area of low signal, though it is well known that the zone of complete necrosis may lie around 3mm inside the edge.

Early assessment of necrosis: verification

In the prostate, the inflammatory reaction and usually the relatively small volume of residual tumor make visualization of residual cancer in the early posttreatment period difficult [3]. A method for delineating necrosis can provide information about technical success and technique effectiveness. As it falls neatly into neither category, we will call such a method *verification*. Especially with ablative techniques, it is hard to imagine how the operator might fully evolve their technique to maximize tumor coverage and minimize collateral damage (to rectum, neurovascular bundles, and sphincter) without the early feedback that verification imaging can provide.

Necrotic tissue changes in elasticity and shows altered proton diffusion. Both MR and ultrasound can be used to measure tissue elasticity and delineate the hardening effect of heating, and consistent changes have been shown in the MR diffusion properties of the prostate both after cryoablation and HIFU. Much more sensitive is the use of techniques that assess perfusion in the treated prostate. CT with intravenous contrast is commonly used after ablation in the liver and kidney, in part because it can be performed in a breath hold, but respiratory motion is much less of a problem in the prostate and MR (and potentially ultrasound) provide superior soft-tissue contrast.

Ultrasound and MRI for assessing necrosis

Ultrasound has the fundamental advantage over CT and MRI that it can delineate blood flow without the need for intravenous contrast. However, the drawback is one of sensitivity: it relies on detection of Doppler shift in vessels and is unlikely to detect small areas of persisting perfusion with slow flow. The sensitivity can be considerably increased with the use of intravenous contrast agents, and this method has been used successfully to delineate the treated volume after HIFU [4]. Some have shown a good correlation between the nonperfused volume on ultrasound and histology at prostatectomy, with ultrasound slightly *underestimating* the volume of necrosis. The MR and ultrasound findings often correlate well (Figure 17.2).

For focal ablation, ultrasound is an attractive technique: it can be performed during the procedure (Figure 17.1) or soon after, potentially allowing dose escalation or retreatment of persistently perfused areas in the

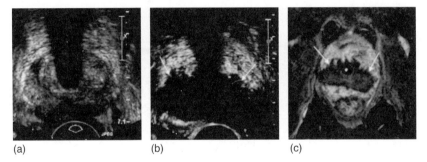

(a)   (b)   (c)

Figure 17.2   Images of a 71-year-old man 1 day after treatment of the whole prostate by HIFU (Ablatherm). (a) A standard transrectal ultrasound image of the prostate. (b) An image after intravenous microbubble contrast (4.8 cc of Sonovue (Bracco, Italy)) (note the central shadowing from the catheter in the urethra). (c) A postcontrast T1-weighted image. Both (b) and (c) show the area of necrosis (arrows), with anterior sparing. (Images courtesy of Dr. O Rouviere.)

same sitting. However, one note of caution in this context is that with photodynamic therapies it may take several hours for progression to full necrosis, so that real, or near-real-time feedback may underestimate coverage.

There are drawbacks on the use of ultrasound, mainly stemming from the relatively poor delineation of the index tumor compared to MRI. If this is not well seen on ultrasound, it may be difficult to assess whether the treatment has covered the tumor, and the need arises for image fusion (whether in the mind of the operator or using a technical solution).

MRI: scanning protocol, appearance after focal treatment, and histological correlates

The T2 signal of the treated prostate is usually heterogenous after ablation, although it may be predominantly low. The T1 signal depends on the amount of hemorrhage and is variable. Neither can accurately delineate necrosis.

To demonstrate nonperfused prostate accurately, intravenous contrast is necessary. Dynamic sequences are usually used for the detection of tumor before treatment, but are not absolutely necessary, and spin echo sequences will suffice after treatment in the early period (Table 17.1). Precontrast sequences are essential because most techniques for focal therapy are likely to produce high-signal hemorrhage, mimicking enhancement – if severe, it may be necessary to generate subtracted images. Although it does not show necrosis well, a T2-weighted high-resolution sequence is important to show the margins of the gland.

The best time for the posttreatment MR has not yet been determined, but for ablative techniques is likely to be less than 5 days after treatment:

Table 17.1 MR sequences used for prostate imaging. Contrast used is 0.1mmol/kg gadoteric acid (Dotarem®; Guerbet, Villepinte, France), given intravenously at 3ml/s. We always perform sequence 1. For scans early (<1 month) after HIFU, *either* sequence 5 or sequences 2 and 6 will adequately delineate necrosis, and we do not perform diffusion weighted imaging. For scans at 6 months or later to detect residual tumour, we perform T2, diffusion-weighted and dynamic contrast-enhanced scans (1, 3, 4 and 5).

	TR	TE	Flip angle/ degrees	Plane	Slice thickness (gap)	Matrix size	Field of view /mm	Time for scan
1. T2 TSE	5170	92	180	axial	3mm (10% gap)	256 × 256	180 × 180	3m 54s each
2. T1 TSE	502	15	150	axial	3mm (10% gap)	256 × 256	200 × 200	2m 44s
3. Diffusion (b values: 0, 150, 500, 1000)	2200	98		axial	5mm	172 × 172	260 × 260	5m 44s (16 averages)
4. Diffusion (b = 1400)	2200	98		axial	5mm	172 × 172	320 × 320	3m 39s (32 averages)
5. VIBE with fat sat	5.61	2.52	15	axial	3mm (20% gap)	192 × 192	260 × 260	7m at least (sequential 16s acquisitions)
6. T1 post contrast fat sat	461	15	150	Axial, coronal	3mm (10% gap)	256 × 256	200 × 200	4m 39s each

in the whole prostate the volume of nonenhancing tissue can decline by around 50% in the first month as involution takes place, and in smaller treated volumes it is possible that this process happens more rapidly.

Appearances after thermal ablation

In the whole prostate, ablation with HIFU is followed by swelling (by up to 50%), lasting up to several weeks, and then a gradual reduction in volume as necrotic tissue is replaced by fibrosis. In our experience, the swelling is less conspicuous after focal therapy and depends on the proportion of the gland treated.

The necrotic tissue is variable on T2-weighted sequences, but seen well after contrast as a nonenhancing, confluent core surrounded by a relatively brightly enhancing rim. The prostate outside the enhancing rim but close to the treatment shows variable change, likely due to a combination of local heating insufficient to cause necrosis and an inflammatory reaction to adjacent necrotic tissue. This often produces moderate reduction in T2 signal and diffuse enhancement, especially conspicuous in the peripheral zone, and potentially lasting many months (Figure 17.3); a pitfall is to report it as suspicious for contralateral tumor.

At this stage, and especially with variable and sometimes florid enhancement, residual tumor is hard to see, but incomplete treatment may still be suspected. There is often ill-defined, "wispy" or linear enhancement at the edge of the treated zone, sometimes only conspicuous on the later postcontrast images. If this enhancement overlaps the tumor seen before treatment, residual disease is likely (Figure 17.3).

Appearances after cryotherapy

No published data exist on the MR appearances after focal cryotherapy, but experience in whole-gland treatment has shown a volume of nonenhancing tissue, with reactive hyperemia in the adjacent tissues, and a "halo" or "penumbra" around the nonenhancing zone. Our limited experience in focal therapy has shown similar effects.

Appearances after PDT

Photodynamic therapy in the prostate is at an early stage, with phase II trials in progress, and there is only one report on posttreatment appearances on MR [5]. After contrast most of the prostate tissue fell into two categories: either nonenhancing or enhancing similarly to pretreatment scans. Nonenhancing islands were often surrounded by relatively normal, enhancing tissue.

Our experience of focal PDT is of well-defined areas of confluent necrosis, often conforming to the shape of the prostate (Figure 17.4), and perhaps with a similar enhancing rim to thermal techniques. However, as in

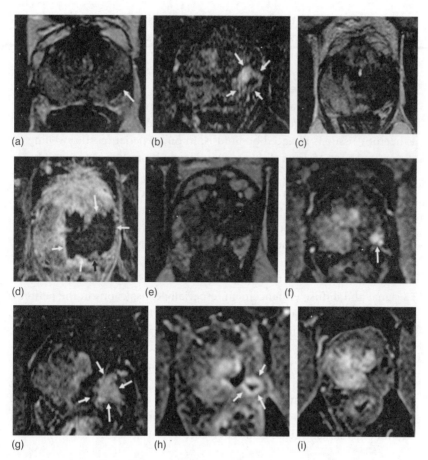

(a)   (b)   (c)

(d)   (e)   (f)

(g)   (h)   (i)

Figure 17.3   Focal ablation in a 68-year-old man. (a, b) T2-weighted and early
contrast-enhanced images showing the tumor in the left-peripheral zone (arrows). (c,
d) T2-weighted and early contrast-enhanced images 1 week after treatment; the
contrast image shows the nonenhancing zone (white arrows) and a small focus of
enhancement just overlapping the site of the original tumor (black arrow). (e, f) The
prostate 6 months after treatment. Note the atrophy of the left hemiprostate and a
small focus of intense early enhancement (arrow). A diffuse blush of enhancement on
the *untreated* side (black arrows) is a common finding and usually reactive rather than
due to disease spread. Biopsies just after this scan were negative for residual disease.
The PSA rose slowly over the next year (reaching 2.8 ng/mL), and a further MRI
showed enlargement of this focus of enhancement ((g), arrows). Further biopsy was
positive for residual disease, and a further targeted HIFU treatment was performed. A
contrast-enhanced scan (h) 3 months later shows the enhancing rim (white arrows)
expected at this stage after HIFU—which may take up to 5 months to resolve—but no
sign of residual disease. Finally, a contrast-enhanced scan 11 months after retreatment
(i) shows no evidence of residual disease. The PSA is stable and a further biopsy has not
yet been performed.

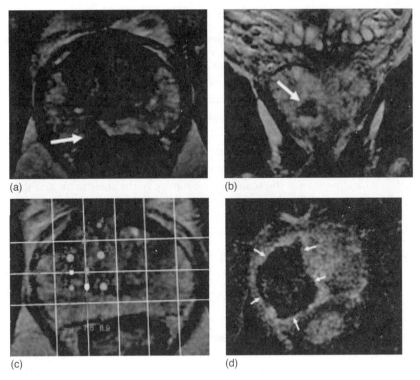

Figure 17.4 Planning and early appearances after focal photodynamic therapy. (a, b) Axial and coronal T2-weighted images, respectively, showing the tumor (white arrow). (c) The treatment planning image, with positions for fiber placement. (d) A postcontrast T1-weighted axial image showing the resulting area of confluent necrosis at 7 days (white arrows). (See Plate 17.4.)

radiotherapy, and in contrast to HIFU (and to a lesser extent cryotherapy), there is little sloughing of necrotic tissue.

Early appearances: histological correlates

The key question to be answered in MR imaging of necrosis is: does lack of enhancement imply nonviable, necrotic tissue? Also, what is the significance of the hyperenhancing rim and how much viable tissue is it likely to contain? This rim is a constant finding in several tissues, including liver, kidney, and brain. In the liver it becomes gradually less conspicuous over 6 months and is seen on both CT and MRI. Within the prostate, it has been shown to occur after laser ablation of benign prostatic hyperplasia as well as HIFU.

Histological evidence in animal models—including rabbit and porcine liver, suggest that the enhancing rim corresponds to an area of inflammation and then fibrosis, with a variable amount of residual, viable tissue.

How much of the rim will be viable after ablation of the prostate in humans remains uncertain.

There is one study of a prototype rotating transurethral ultrasound ablative device in dog prostates that has interesting results. In this study, the necrosis at histology is complete centrally around the device in the urethra. A line drawn around the nonenhancing area at contrast-enhanced MR lies *within* a line drawn at the junction of complete and incomplete necrosis on histology: in other words, the nonenhancing tissue always indicated complete necrosis [6]. The implication from this and other studies is likely to be that a variable amount of the rim contains viable tissue (depending on the organ being scanned, the nature of the treatment, and the interval before the scan), and the only reliably necrotic area at MR is that which does not enhance.

Prognostic value of early MR

Tumor treatment

There is virtually no published work looking at the prognostic value of early MRI in focal therapy, though there is a small amount of work correlating early MR appearances with intermediate measures of outcome after whole-gland cryotherapy and HIFU. Donnelly et al. examined the appearance of the prostate at contrast-enhanced MR 3 weeks after cryotherapy and correlated it with PSA levels and the result of a transrectal biopsy at 6 months [7]. To their surprise, they found no significant correlation of imaging scores (related to persisting enhancing tissue) with the presence of viable prostate or tumor at future biopsy, although they did (not surprisingly) note a correlation between PSA level and the likelihood of residual disease. In contrast, we have found different results in a small group of 13 patients who underwent contrast-enhanced MR less than 1 month after whole-gland HIFU: those with the most enhancing prostatic tissue on the early scan were most likely to have residual tumor at 6-month biopsy [3].

Complications

The significance of rectal wall necrosis depends critically on whether there has been previous radiotherapy. Rectal fistula is now almost unheard of in primary HIFU and cryotherapy, and in our experience a segment of nonenhancing rectal wall, even if apparently complete, usually does not lead to fistula. However, in patients who have undergone external beam radiotherapy the finding is more ominous. If there has also been brachytherapy, fistulation is likely, but often takes several months to occur (Figure 17.5). Although rectal fistulation may be suspected on early imaging, it usually presents several weeks or more after treatment, and ultimately requires

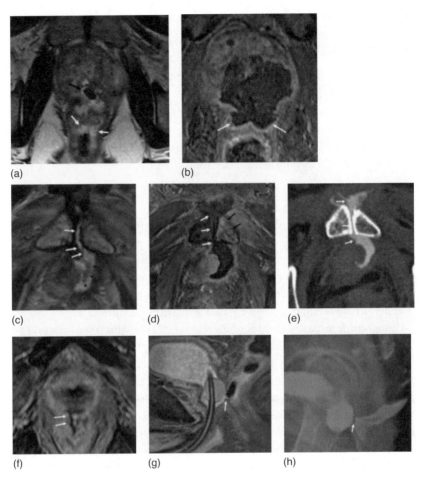

(a)   (b)

(c)   (d)   (e)

(f)   (g)   (h)

Figure 17.5   Three examples of fistulation. In the first patient, focal treatment
resulted in signal change in the rectal wall (white arrow on the T2-weighted image—
(a)), considerable posterior extraprostatic necrosis—seen best on the postcontrast image
(white arrows in (b)) and an air bubble within the prostate (black arrow in (a)).
Although there were symptoms of a prostatorectal fistula, they subsequently resolved
and a urethrogram did not show a leak. Such resolution is rare even if there has not
been previous radiotherapy. (c–e) T2-weighted, T1 postcontrast, and CT (10 minutes
after iv contrast) images, respectively, of an anterior fistula developing 6 months after
left hemi-HIFU in a patient who had previously undergone brachytherapy and external
beam radiotherapy. The white arrows in each case show the fistulating urine. Note the
abnormal enhancement in the adjacent symphisis (black arrow, (d)). Note also the
persisting, nonenhancing debris in the treated zone (black arrowheads, (c))—a
common finding after radiotherapy. Finally, (f) and (g) are T1-weighted and STIR
images in a patient who underwent two HIFU treatments for recurrent prostate cancer
after radiotherapy. The fistula is seen as a track of nonenhancement, and high signal
extending across a thinned rectal wall on STIR (white arrows)—note the foley catheter
in the prostatic fossa. It was confirmed on urethrogram (h), and required a salvage
prostatectomy.

reconstructive surgery. The track can be seen as an area of high signal on T2 or STIR images, or a persisting linear focus of reduced enhancement (from edema and fluid in the track).

Findings at 2–5 months

Just as it may take several months for the PSA to stabilize, or reach nadir level, after prostate ablation, it takes some time for the appearances to stabilize after HIFU: usually around 6 months after treatment of the whole gland and sometimes a little less after focal therapy.

Appearances at 6 months

In most cases of primary ablation, the visible nonenhancing necrotic material has been resorbed by 6 months, although this process may take much longer if there has been previous radiotherapy, where (especially if recurrence is not suspected) it may be best to wait 9–12 months before imaging. The treated prostate becomes markedly smaller and is replaced by fibrosis of generally low signal on T2-weighted sequences (Figure 17.3)

Though tumor may sometimes be visible on T2-weighted sequences, recurrent disease will best be seen as an enhancing focus early after intravenous contrast. If the whole prostate has been ablated, such a focus is often seen on a background of fibrosis, which enhances less and more slowly than tumor. In focal therapy, the situation is slightly more complicated: especially if there are narrow margins, there may be adjacent enhancing prostate, and this may show some persisting inflammation. Even so, tumor will usually show early-peaking, often intense enhancement. For this reason, we recommend dynamic sequences for imaging at >6 months, with a time resolution of 15 seconds or better, to enable characterization of enhancement curves in difficult cases (Table 17.1) (Figure 17.6). Others have also used diffusion-weighted imaging, finding high signal on diffusion-weighted images with a b-value of 1000 s/mm^2 and restriction on an ADC map.

After cryotherapy, MR shows loss of zonal anatomy on T2 sequences after whole-gland treatment, with the formation of a "thick, fibrous capsule" around the prostate, although appearances after contrast enhancement have not been described.

Diffuse reduction in gland size, reduced signal, and loss of zonal differentiation has been described after brachytherapy, and is similar to changes seen after treatment of the whole gland by external beam radiotherapy; no data has been published on the appearance of residual disease but we have noted intense, early enhancement in several patients, similar to the appearance of recurrent disease after external beam radiotherapy (Figure 17.7).

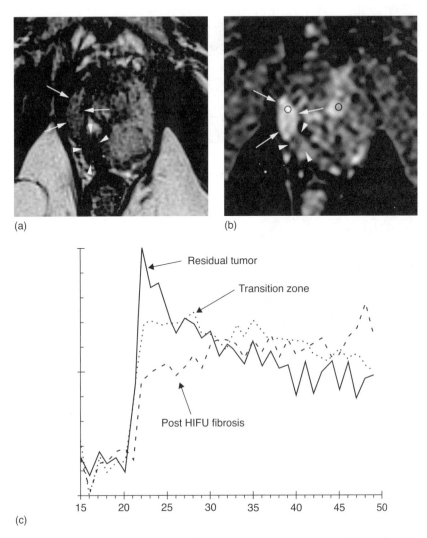

Figure 17.6 Residual disease 6 months after HIFU (white arrow, (a and b)) and corresponding enhancement curves (c). Tumor enhances early, and intensely, relative to fibrotic, treated prostate (white arrowheads (a and b)), and the untreated half of the gland.

Six months onward: detecting residual disease and monitoring for recurrence

Imaging has a potentially important role to play in the monitoring of patients after focal therapy, and one that may not be fully appreciated by most urologists. Data already exist to suggest that PSA and contrast-enhanced MR are of similar sensitivity for the detection of residual disease after *whole-gland* ablation, and there is little doubt that PSA will be a less

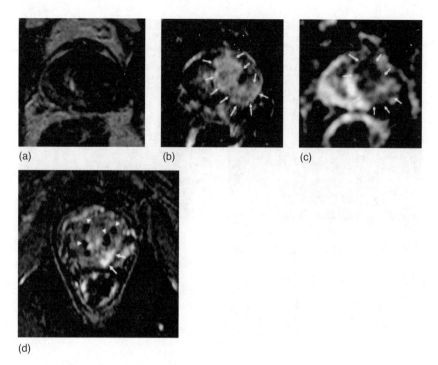

(a) (b) (c)

(d)

Figure 17.7 Two examples of recurrent disease after radiotherapy. (a, b, c) T2-weighted, contrast-enhanced, and diffusion-weighted (ADC) scans, respectively, from the same patient with a rising PSA several years after radiotherapy. Note that on T2 the whole gland is low in signal and tumor difficult to distinguish. It is well seen after contrast and on the diffusion sequences as an area of restriction (white arrows). (d) An early postcontrast scan in a different patient after brachytherapy (note the areas of susceptibility artefact from the seeds, arrowheads) showing a smaller focus of tumor (white arrow).

sensitive test when unpredictable production from untreated prostate is added to the equation. Furthermore, although in most patients undergoing focal therapy the incidence of nodal and metastatic disease is likely to be low, a fundamental limit to the performance of PSA is that rises may be due to local recurrence or metastatic spread.

Six months and later: histological correlation and prognostic information

There are as yet no published studies looking at the ability of imaging to detect residual disease after focal treatment, so we will describe those for the different whole-gland treatments. How much the additional complexity of adjacent, untreated or partly treated prostate in focal therapy will complicate detection of residual disease is uncertain.

There are several published series examining the ability of MR to detect residual disease after whole-gland HIFU. The largest is a series of 27 patients, analyzed by sextant, where the results of dynamic contrast-enhanced scans were compared with T2 and diffusion-weighted images. The dynamic contrast sequences showed better sensitivity (mean sensitivity 83%, specificity 66%) than the T2 plus diffusion-weighted images, but the latter had better specificity (mean sensitivity 66%, specificity 76%) [8].

Our group has found that inexperienced observers can achieve a sensitivity of 75% and specificity of 76% for the detection of disease recurrence in the whole gland [9], with an area under the receiver operating characteristic curve similar to that for PSA. Finally, recent evidence from Rouviere et al. shows that biopsies targeted to areas of suspicion for recurrence on MR are much more likely to be positive than standard cores, with 22% of recurrences only found on MR-directed cores, although specificity was not high, and residual prostate tissue was often identified as suspicious [10].

The combination of T2 weighted sequences and spectroscopy has been examined in a group of 13 patients. Although the numbers are too small for meaningful estimates of sensitivity and specificity, an important finding was that MR spectroscopy was suitable for analysis *in only 3 out of the 10 patients* who had partial necrosis [11].

Cryotherapy: Parivar et al. have assessed the performance of magnetic resonance spectroscopy for the detection of residual disease after cryotherapy in a series of 25 patients, 5 of whom had an undetectable PSA several months after treatment [12]. MR spectroscopy correctly identified 8 patients with residual disease, but there were false positives (if biopsy was defined as the gold standard) in 5 out of 17 patients. There is currently no published data assessing the use of gadolinium-based contrast after cryotherapy.

Imaging after brachytherapy and radiotherapy: No studies have assessed the ability to detect residual disease after brachytherapy, but recurrent tumor after external beam radiotherapy to the whole gland can be detected with a sensitivity of 68% and specificity over 90% using T2 sequences alone, while the addition of spectroscopy improved sensitivity a little but at the cost of a marked increase in false positives [13]. Dynamic contrast enhancement and diffusion-weighted imaging clearly improve detection [14,15] with combined diffusion and dynamic contrast enhancement showing improved performance beyond each sequence on its own [16,17]. We have also successfully detected tumor after brachytherapy as intense foci of enhancement seen in between the signal voids that result from seeds on gradient-echo sequences (Figure 17.7).

Summary

Focal therapy is more exacting than treatment of the whole prostate for many reasons, many of which strengthen the case for imaging after the procedure. Firstly, we are using a set of technologies for focal ablation that are relatively untested in this application, and early (*verification*) posttreatment imaging has the unique potential to provide feedback to the operator (and to the device developer) about the lesions being produced, and their accuracy. Secondly, PSA becomes a less attractive modality for follow-up as the proportion of prostate treated decreases, because of unpredictable production from residual prostate. One alternative is repeat biopsies for follow up, but this has practical and safety implications if focal therapy were widely adopted. A lifetime of biopsies may not be relished by the patient, and it is worth remembering that biopsy will miss a considerable number of small local recurrences. Finally, the ability of MR to define the anatomical location of recurrent disease is no less important in planning retreatment than in the primary therapy: the advantages of *focal* retreatment for recurrence are likely to mirror those of focal therapy in general.

References

1. Goldberg SN, et al. Image-guided tumor ablation: standardization of terminology and reporting criteria. *J Vasc Interv Radiol* 2005;16: 765–778.
2. Atri M, et al. Contrast-enhanced ultrasonography for real-time monitoring of interstitial laser thermal therapy in the focal treatment of prostate cancer. *Can Urol Assoc J* 2009;3: 125–130.
3. Kirkham APS, Emberton M, Hoh IM. et al. MR imaging of prostate after treatment with high-intensity focused ultrasound. *Radiology* 2008;246: 833.
4. Rouviere O, et al. Transrectal HIFU ablation of prostate cancer: assessment of tissue destruction with contrast-enhanced ultrasound. *Eur Urol Suppl* 2009;8: 356.
5. Haider MA, et al. Prostate gland: MR imaging appearance after vascular targeted photodynamic therapy with palladium-bacteriopheophorbide. *Radiology* 2007;244: 196–204.
6. Boyes A, et al. Prostate Tissue Analysis Immediately Following Magnetic Resonance Imaging Guided Transurethral Ultrasound Thermal Therapy. *J Urol* 2007;178: 1080–1085.
7. Donnelly SE, et al. Prostate cancer: gadolinium-enhanced MR imaging at 3 weeks compared with needle biopsy at 6 months after cryoablation. *Radiology* 2004;232: 830–833.
8. Kim C, et al. MRI Techniques for Prediction of Local Tumor Progression After High-Intensity Focused Ultrasonic Ablation of Prostate Cancer. *American J Roentgenol* 2008;190: 1180–1186.
9. Kirkham A, et al. The value of Magnetic resonance imaging and PSA in detecting recurrence after high intensity focused ultrasound. *Eur Urol Suppl* 2009;8: 322.

10. Rouviere O, et al. Prostate cancer transrectal HIFU ablation: detection of local recurrences with MRI. *Eur Urol Suppl* 2009;8: 322.

11. Cirillo S, et al. Endorectal magnetic resonance imaging and magnetic resonance spectroscopy to monitor the prostate for residual disease or local cancer recurrence after transrectal high-intensity focused ultrasound. *BJUInt* 2008;102: 452–458.

12. Parivar F, et al. Detection of locally recurrent prostate cancer after cryosurgery: evaluation by transrectal ultrasound, magnetic resonance imaging, and three-dimensional proton magnetic resonance spectroscopy. *Urology* 1996;48: 594–599.

13. Pucar D, et al. Prostate cancer: correlation of MR imaging and MR spectroscopy with pathologic findings after radiation therapy-initial experience. *Radiology* 2005;236: 545–553.

14. Haider MA, et al. Dynamic contrast-enhanced magnetic resonance imaging for localization of recurrent prostate cancer after external beam radiotherapy. *IJRBOP* 2008;70: 425–430.

15. Kim CK, et al. Prediction of locally recurrent prostate cancer after radiation therapy: incremental value of 3T diffusion-weighted MRI. *J Magn Reson Imaging* 2009;29: 391–397.

16. Kim C, et al. Prostate MR imaging at 3T using a phased-arrayed coil in predicting locally recurrent prostate cancer after radiation therapy: preliminary experience. *Abdom Imaging* 2010;35(2): 246–252.

17. Arumainayagam N, et al. Accuracy of multiparametric magnetic resonance imaging in detecting recurrent prostate cancer after radiotherapy. *BJUInt* 2010; 106(7): 991–997.

CHAPTER 18

Evaluating Focal Therapy: Future Perspectives

Hashim U. Ahmed MRCS BM BCh BA(Hons)[1] and Mark Emberton FRCS (Urol) FRCS MD MBBS BSc[1,2]

[1]Division of Surgery and Interventional Sciences, University College London, London, UK
[2]NIHR UCL/UCH Comprehensive Biomedical Research Centre, London, UK

Introduction

There is a clear need to evaluate focal therapy in order to measure medium to long-term cancer control rates within a randomized controlled trial (RCT). We propose that this strategy incorporates the principles based on the United Kingdom's Medical Research Council guidelines for evaluating complex interventions, and closely reflecting the IDEAL (Innovation, Development, Exploration, Assessment, Long-term) guidelines for assessing surgical innovations.

RCTs in which surgery is compared to conservative measures can be difficult to recruit. Trials need to be broad in entry criteria and pragmatic in design so that surgeon and patient equipoise is reflected and recruitment and external validity improved. Pragmatic trials overcome issues related to equipoise and general applicability by reflecting decisions, treatment options, follow-up, and outcome measures that fall within standard clinical practice.

A pragmatic design could incorporate the following factors:

1 Men with low- to intermediate-risk disease.
2 Cancer localized by techniques that meet physician/patient preference.
3 Interventions that reflect local expertise (cryotherapy, HIFU, brachytherapy).
4 Comparators that include standard of care (active surveillance or radical therapy) in order to reflect individual physician/patient equipoise.

There is little consensus on the optimal outcomes to use in an RCT other than the rate of metastatic disease/mortality, which requires trials

---

Focal Therapy in Prostate Cancer, First Edition. Edited by Hashim U Ahmed, Manit Arya, Peter Carroll and Mark Emberton.
© 2012 Blackwell Publishing Ltd. Published 2012 by Blackwell Publishing Ltd.

with very large numbers, huge resource, and over 10–15 years follow-up. Although it should be the intention to follow-up men long term, outcomes such as need for hormonal therapy and impact on quality of life may allow novel interventions in prostate cancer to be evaluated without large resources and infrastructure in order to benefit patients early.

Pragmatic and adaptive trial design

RCTs in which surgery is compared to conservative measures can be difficult to recruit [1]. In addition, many have argued that as currently conducted, RCTs are inefficient, complex, time-consuming, expensive, and report outcomes that have little relevance at the time of reporting [2].

Randomized trials in prostate cancer that began over a decade ago, such as PIVOT [3], ProTect, and the Scandinavian SPCG-4 trial have been successful in recruitment, but have required a large infrastructure and much expense to conduct and complete. Indeed, Pivot required 52 centers that screened over 13,000 men, of which 5000 met entry criteria and 731 were eventually randomized. In the case of ProTect, dedicated nursing staff to counsel patients regarding randomization were needed [4]. However, more recently randomized trial designs in prostate cancer have had problems in recruitment (Sabre, ProStart, SPIRIT, Canadian randomized trial comparing external beam radiotherapy with cryosurgery) [5, 6].

The need for trials to be efficient, cost effective, and future-proof by capitalizing on existing resource and having a pragmatic and adaptive approach to design is key to delivering answers to healthcare services on comparative effectiveness of novel interventions in a timely fashion. Necessary attributes of such trials comprise broad entry criteria that are representative of routine practice and a pragmatic design that mimics real-life practice as much as is possible. One of the main barriers to recruitment is that the equipoise of patients considering enrollment and clinicians advising them does not mirror the equipoise in those who designed the study [7]. Pragmatic trials that have an adaptive approach overcome some of the issues related to external validity and equipoise by attempting to reflect decisions, treatment options, follow-up, and outcome measures that fall within standard clinical practice. In addition, a pragmatic design must be open to incorporating worthy novel interventions during the lifetime of the trial. This "dynamic learning adaptive" feature improves timeliness and clinical relevance of trial results.

The following sections outline the options that are available in choosing the patient population, the exact intervention, comparator and outcome measures from an explanatory RCT, and a pragmatic and adaptive design.

Population

Risk category

Explanatory
Low- to intermediate-risk prostate cancer (PSA $\leq$ 15 ng/mL, Gleason $\leq$ 7, T1–T2cN0M0)

Pragmatic
No restrictions on risk category, but local preference (physician/patient) determines entry into trial

Intervention

Disease localization

Explanatory
The exact mode of disease localization is set in the protocol with only one of the localization strategies selected to ensure standardization across all sites.

Pragmatic
The exact mode of disease localization can be determined by local preference and incorporate novel imaging tools as and when they become available. These would include any or a number of the following:
1 Multiparametric (mp)-MRI +/− biopsy
2 mpMRI + template mapping biopsies
3 Template biopsies alone
4 Ultrasound tissue characterization +/− biopsy
5 Imaging alone

Timing of disease localization

Explanatory
Disease localization will be used to determine suitability for focal therapy conducted prior to randomization so that men who are deemed unsuitable for focal therapy are not selected for randomization. However, such a proposal will exclude a group that is likely to have a higher burden and risk of disease (work-up bias). The requirement for patients interested in the trial to undergo two tests prior to randomization that are currently not part of standard care has a cost and healthcare burden.

Pragmatic

Disease localization is carried out after randomization, effectively becoming part of the focal therapy strategy. This would reduce selection bias. An intention-to-treat analysis would ensure that those deemed unsuitable for focal therapy after randomization are included in the focal therapy arm.

Ablative technology

Explanatory

This would control the modality of ablation in order to ensure standardization. This would limit the number of centers and exclude other future ablative technologies that could deliver focal therapy. However, standardization of the intervention and ensuring centers are beyond learning curves ensures that focal therapy is tested in an optimal setting so as to prevent a false negative result from the RCT.

Pragmatic

All approved ablative technologies demonstrating ability to ablate in a focal manner – the trial therefore testing the concept of focal therapy, not the technology. At the moment, HIFU and cryotherapy conform closely to the desired attributes and have the added advantage that the skills required to deliver the intervention in a quality assured manner are already in place in a number of centers in Europe. Both ablative interventions could be incorporated into one trial protocol essentially allowing site-specific ablation; the exact intervention within the focal therapy arm will be determined by the imaging and histopathological localization and the particular expertise of a center. Other treatments such as photodynamic therapy, photothermal therapy, radio-frequency ablation, injectables, and electroporation could all be incorporated as and when they demonstrate early effectiveness within prospective trials incorporating appropriate histological endpoints.

Strategy of ablation

Explanatory

The untreated areas will have absence of any cancer on template biopsies. This will reduce the external validity of the findings by incorporating unknown selection bias.

Pragmatic

The untreated areas will have absence of clinically significant cancer on whichever localization strategy is used (absence of Gleason pattern 4 and high burden cancer) [8]. This reflects current uncertainty about what constitutes significant cancer. It is also likely that the side, which is deemed negative on template-mapping biopsies harbors low volume low-grade disease that, by random error due to the 5-mm spacing of the sampling, was simply missed. The pragmatic design acknowledges and embraces this known error by incorporating a threshold of clinical significance based on grade and burden.

Comparators

Explanatory

This will limit the comparator arm to either active surveillance or whole-gland therapy, possibly limiting the latter to radiotherapy or surgery in order to standardize the comparator. This will also ensure outcome measures more straightforward to measure.

Pragmatic

The comparator arm will be standard care (Figure 18.1). Both active surveillance and radical therapy are regarded as current standard care for men with low- to –intermediate-risk prostate cancer, dependent on other factors such a comorbidity, age, and life expectancy. There is currently no consensus on whether focal therapy is an alternative to active surveillance or radical therapies, although it is likely that it could serve as an alternative to both. Men and their physicians will choose the treatment, surveillance, or whole-gland therapy (surgery, radiotherapy) that they wish to have if randomized to standard care. For example, those men and physicians who favor active surveillance, an alternative therapy that offers a low side effect profile treatment for the cancer with reduced rates of progression or intervention may be appealing. On the contrary, for those men and physicians who favor some form of treatment and would normally choose whole-gland therapy, may find an alternative that offers treatment for the cancer with a low side-effect profile equally appealing.

Effectively, this will permit the patient/clinician to choose the strategy in the comparator arm after randomization. For example, if it was felt that it would not be in the patient's best interest to be managed with active surveillance because of some adverse features of the pathology, then they would choose surgery or radiotherapy. Equally, if a particular man wished to avoid an aspect of whole-gland therapy but would accept surveillance or focal therapy, he would opt for active surveillance in the comparator arm. Such a design more closely represents patient/physician equipoise rather than offering a single randomization that either or both clinician and patient are not comfortable with. Second, criteria for inclusion are less restrictive. Put together, these elements will not only facilitate recruitment but also represent real-life decision-making.

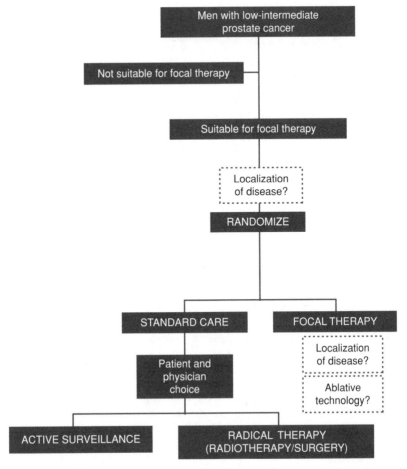

Figure 18.1   Flow diagram demonstrating key features of a pragmatic, dynamic adaptive randomized controlled clinical trial assessing focal therapy in prostate cancer.

Outcomes

Explanatory

1 The rate of metastases and cancer-related mortality
2 Cost effectiveness

Pragmatic

1 The transition in health states (these will be functional health states and cancer health states and will be defined by patients)
2 The rate of additional systemic therapy (with rate of metastases and cancer-related mortality incorporated into Phase IV or registry follow-up linked to national mortality statistical databases)
3 Cost effectiveness and cost-utility

The first pragmatic outcome relates to treatment related side effects and can be relatively well captured using validated questionnaires. These are principally directed at genitourinary and bowel-associated outcomes and have been used in the evaluation of all the interventions under consideration. The second pragmatic outcome relates to effectiveness of cancer control. If the rate of prostate cancer-related deaths were used some 10–15 years would have to pass before sufficient deaths were accrued to make comparisons meaningful with a trial that would require approximately 2000 patients. The prolonged recruitment period with meaningful outcomes reported only 15–20 years later is likely to mean the results will not be timely at the point of reporting. Indeed, due to the very fact that the event rate in mortality is low demonstrates the need to assess new therapies that potentially carry fewer side effects in a short space of time, so that they can be made available in clinical practice to address the large overtreatment burden. Nonetheless, any new therapy must at the same time demonstrate effectiveness of cancer control to ensure it is a safe approach. Therefore, the use of additional systemic therapy could be regarded as the only acceptable outcome measure that would cover focal therapy and standard care.

If the PRECIS (pragmatic-explanatory continuum indicator summary) approach is used and if most of elements of the pragmatic design were adopted, the following pragmatogram would be drawn (Figure 18.2).

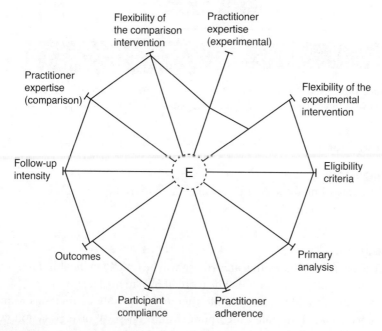

Figure 18.2   A "pragmatogram" outlining the PRECIS features of the trial we suggest in this chapter.

Some degree of quality control of centers conducting focal therapy will be necessary, hence the loss of pragmatic conduct in this particular field.

Conclusion

The future of focal therapy as a strategy in the therapeutic armamentarium of physicians treating men with prostate cancer is unknown. However, what is clear is the need for robust study designs so that if men are to benefit from a potentially effective treatment that carries minimal impact on function, guideline committees and regulatory authorities are convinced by outcomes from such trials. Equally, it is important that new randomized studies are pragmatic so that they reflect true decision-making in the clinic with few hurdles to entry, so that randomized studies in focal therapy recruit and report in a timely fashion to benefit men with prostate cancer.

References

1. Brubaker L, et al. Challenges in designing a pragmatic clinical trial: the mixed incontinence - medical or surgical approach (MIMOSA) trial experience. *Clin Trials* 2009;6(4): 355–364.
2. Luce BR, et al. Rethinking randomized clinical trials for comparative effectiveness research: the need for transformational change. *Ann Intern Med* 2009;151(3): 206–209.
3. Wilt TJ, et al. The Prostate cancer Intervention Versus Observation Trial:VA/NCI/ AHRQ Cooperative Studies Program #407 (PIVOT): design and baseline results of a randomized controlled trial comparing radical prostatectomy to watchful waiting for men with clinically localized prostate cancer. *Contemp Clin Trials* 2009;30(1): 81–87.
4. Donovan JL et al; ProtecT Study Group. Who can best recruit to randomized trials? Randomized trial comparing surgeons and nurses recruiting patients to a trial of treatments for localized prostate cancer (the ProtecT study). *J Clin Epidemiol* 2003;56(7): 605–609.
5. Donnelly BJ, et al. A randomized trial of external beam radiotherapy versus cryoablation in patients with localized prostate cancer. *Cancer* 2010;116(2): 323–330.
6. Crook JM, et al. Comparison of Health-Related Quality of Life 5 Years After SPIRIT: Surgical Prostatectomy Versus Interstitial Radiation Intervention Trial. *J Clin Oncol* 2011;29(4): 362–368.
7. Tunis SR, et al. Practical clinical trials: increasing the value of clinical research for decision making in clinical and health policy. *JAMA* 2003;290: 1624–1632.
8. Ahmed HU. The index lesion and the origin of prostate cancer. *N Engl J Med* 2009; 361(17): 1704–1706.

Index

Note: Page numbers with italicized *f*'s and *t*'s refer to figures and tables, respectively.

Focal Therapy in Prostate Cancer, First Edition. Edited by Hashim U Ahmed, Manit Arya,
Peter Carroll and Mark Emberton.
© 2012 Blackwell Publishing Ltd. Published 2012 by Blackwell Publishing Ltd.